Recreate Your Health One Year to a New You

DR. RACHEL BROOKS

Disclaimer-

The procedures described in this book are not meant to diagnose or treat any condition. The information presented in this book has been compiled from my clinical experience and research. It is offered as a view of the relationship between diet, exercise, emotions, and health. This book simply contains supportive and palliative protocols to follow for a better quality of life.

This book is intended solely to help you make better judgements concerning your long-term health goals. If you are experiencing health problems, you should consult a qualified physician immediately. Remember early examination and detection are important to successful treatment of all diseases.

Table of Contents

Letter To The Reader 1

Why Are You Here 3

What Is Health? 13

Month 1 Chiropractic, Optimal Digestion, and Journaling 24

Month 2 Inflammation, Movement, and Being Social 42

Month 3 Team Sports, Gluten, and Accountability 56

Month 4 Sugar, High Intensity Interval Training, and Community 73

Month 5 Detoxification, Slowing Down, and Getting Outdoors 88

Month 6 Light Therapy, Paleo Lifestyle, and Posture 103

Month 7 Yoga, Functional Medicine, and Meditation 121

Month 8 Leaky Gut, Gut-Brain Barrier, and How Pain Works 137

Month 9 Massage, Household Chemicals, and Putting Yourself First ... 153

Month 10 Ketogenic Diet, Weight Loss, and Mindset 165

Month 11 Drugs, Core Work, and Seeking Help 184

Month 12 Intermittent Fasting, Acupuncture, and Personal Developement 197

Bonus Month: Balancing Macros, Squats, and Sleep 212

The Journey Beyond 223

Appendix 228

Letter To The Reader

Dear Reader,

The purpose of this book is to provide you with the tools that will help you become the your picture of health. The biggest problem with most wellness journeys is that we expect a drastic transformation in 30 days. However, transformative changes take months to years. My intention is that this book provides 12 steps or 12 months of instruction on how to create a life of fitness and wellbeing. I mean for you to find which programs work for you and which do not. Everyone has differing body physiology. You will hopefully find a few steps that truly make a difference in your life and those are the ones to stick to in the long term. If one month does not resonate with you or it does not provide any benefit, simply recognize it as a step along your journey and move on to the next chapter.

I also encourage you to stay within a chapter for more than one month if it really produces a change in your life. Think of this journey as an accumulation of tools to create a better life. Stick to the tools that work for you as you progress. If you find a lifestyle change that drastically benefits you, don't ditch it because the next chapter has a different plan.

Each chapter is structured on a combination of information and assignments. I will give you a background of information on each topic, and then add assignments related to it. There will be instructions based on each angle of the triad of health. The Triad of health will be discussed later, but for simplicity, it is the concept that health involves chemical, structural, and mental aspects. We are trying to create wellbeing in all three so all three will be addressed in each chapter.

I have attempted to structure your progress in the order in which I discovered my own health potential. I believe I have gotten as far as I have because I gradually added things. I did not just wake up one day and find myself a paleo, cross fitting, alternatively minded chiropractor. It was a journey; a journey that I will always travel. I will always be seeking better health. If you do not aspire to be better, you tend to gradually get worse instead. That is just life. I am not saying to never think you are good enough. I am not saying to hate your body. I am not saying to be perfect all the time. I am saying; always aspire to be better than you were yesterday.

So please, enjoy your journey. Embrace the fact that it will be different from anyone else's. Strive to find the wonderful intelligent doctor that lives within you. Celebrate every victory. Be the best version of you!

Wishing you the best in health,

Dr. Rachel

Why Are You Here

Have you ever aspired to be the person on the cover of some fitness magazine? The one with flat abs, an awesome spouse, time to go on vacation, surfs every day, eats healthy for a living, and just overall seems like they have their shit together? You envy their life. You are possibly sitting in the middle of farm country, hiding behind your excuses. I mean, we can't all live near the beach in Cali. Or maybe you actually live in an area with all the best options but they are too expensive or maybe you feel out of place in those crowds. You feel too fat to put yourself in a workout class of fit people. You don't know where to start to even try to achieve the Cali-Surfer-Perfect Life, the picture of health.

There is accurate and free information out there thanks to Google. You can read how to exercise right, eat right, see doctors, and keep your blood work in tune, but, where the hell do you start? With the internet, you can read up on how every lifestyle change can heal you or harm you. Eat fat, don't eat fat. Go vegan, vegan is bad. Lower your cholesterol, cholesterol is needed. Eggs are healthy, eggs will kill you. Exercise, but do not exercise too much. What is true? It is hard to filter through what is important and what is not. Usually, the amount of info is just so overwhelming, you quit before you even start.

Equally challenging is figuring out how to make your life changes manageable. Which program is right for you? It's hard to put $300 out for some supplement program that may not help you at all. You also do not want to make life altering changes without some sort of guarantee on results. You are afraid to waste your time, resources and motivation on just another wellness scheme.

The problem with most "get healthy quick schemes" is that they do work, but have no follow up plan. I have had a number of patients that do a 21 day cleanse or 30 days without sugar. They generally feel awesome. They get on the "New Year, New You" bandwagon and go all in with intense motivation. They eat their way out of pain, they lose a little weight, but halfway through February, they are back to their normal lifestyle and are gradually slipping downhill again. A general rule to think about is this: if you are not moving forward, you are sliding backwards. If you are just going on "Maintenance plans," you are not moving forward. You are getting too comfortable with your current lifestyle, and comfort is the enemy of progress.

This book is designed to give you a minimum 12 months of goals and new protocols to follow. However, this can definitely take a bit longer if that is what's right for you. Some people are what I call "all in" people and some are "step by step" people. Know who you are. This book is an accelerated "step by step" but I am sure the "all in" people will try to cram it in quicker. I wrote this book in congruence with my own search for wellness. It took me years to get through each concept. I am hoping to help you reach your best health faster than I did. Regardless of timing, the main concept will be the same. The concept is constant upward progress, always pushing your limits, setting new goals, and making incremental changes to reach them. We will also be helping you understand WHY you are making the changes. In my practice, I find you are more likely to stick to a guideline or health principle if you understand the physiology behind it. I would like to help you understand your body. Think of this book as a user's guide for your body. Find what motivates you, changes you, and benefits you.

What motivates you?

Most people's goals are weight driven. I am here to tell you, you need to change that. You need to find a WHY. Why do you want to change, why do you want to reach your goal, why do you want to get healthy? Don't get me wrong weight loss is usually a part of any goal. For example, if my goal is to keep up with my husband hiking on vacation, I may need to slim down a bit. If you want off heart medications, often weight loss is required. Keeping up with grandkids, weight loss required. However, if you want weight loss just to look good, that is a purely superficial goal and you will likely lose because of this. You need to make your WHY bigger. A good example could be: I want to lose weight, get fit and be healthy to set an example for my kids. I do not want my kids to struggle with their health and weight as I have so I want to do the right things early in their development.

I am going to be brutally honest here, even if you are totally miserable health wise, like you cannot get through the grocery store without a scooter, you sleep in a recliner because lying flat hurts too much, your relationship is dying because your health has deteriorated so far; you will not reach your goals or change your life if your WHY is simply that you are sick of being miserable. Sometimes, rock bottom isn't even a strong enough motivator for change. Most people would need to have a better WHY. Another example could be: I want to get healthy so I can rekindle my relationship with my husband. I want us to stay together and be happy and my health is preventing that. Health puts a huge weight on a relationship, pun intended. Having health practices that are in sync can be more important than being the same religion in a relationship. Oftentimes, people wait too long to realize this and they suffer. Many people, after a divorce, go through some crazy health transformation.

(Because being alone is a big enough WHY). If they would have made their relationship a big enough why, they would have undergone this transformation pre-divorce and maybe saved their marriage. Relationships do not work if the healthy person feels that they are pulling the dead weight of their lazy gross partner. Obviously, there are some circumstances where health complications are unexpected and traumatic, and spouses really step it up to care for the other. That is still really taxing on a spouse though, isn't it? Even if is it something that could not be prevented? Now imagine the health problem could have been avoided, you are automatically irritated with them. This goes for relationships beyond just husband-wife as well. <u>Being unhealthy is not a purely physical problem. It affects all aspects of your life. It affects your job performance, relationships, energy, productivity, household, and more.</u> After that extended explanation, I hope you can see that my point is to make your WHY about more than just your physique. Make it about maintaining a better quality of life!

Keeping the concept of WHY in mind, this book is going to help you implement simple additions that can make a huge difference in your overall health. Goals and accomplishments must be perceived as being doable or we aren't going to even attempt them. The processes discussed in this book will be full of easy, doable processes that can make a world of a difference in your life, and make achieving your goals less intimidating.

We unfortunately believe that we can change our lives overnight. The truth is that we can change our *mind* overnight, but our body doesn't change that quickly. This is because whatever it was that created the condition of our body didn't happen overnight or even in one or two weeks; it took a lifetime. So if you want to change your health for good, you must look at the healing factor differently. Look at it as an ongoing process that you begin today. For example, it takes years to gain 50 lbs., it will likely take more than 6 months to lose it, right? The same concept applies to acquiring and then healing other maladies.

What you need to do to get something out of this book is to begin by opening your mind. They say the mind is like a parachute, and it won't work if it's not opened. You must have an open mind to try out new ideas, especially those actions that may not be as widely accepted by the mainstream population. Remember, comfort is the enemy of progress. Some assignments may be uncomfortable at first but that is where transformation occurs. Life begins at the end of your comfort zone, so step out of that circle.

We all fear change. Yet we continue on the path that has brought us to the poor physical condition that we now experience. Somehow we imagine in our minds that even staying on the same path can yield different results than the last time we started down it. That is the definition of insanity. You must transform your fear into curiosity and courage. Curiosity might very well be the help you need to bridge the gap from where you are to where you can be. Be curious with trying new things. Have the courage to find out just how well you can feel, and the number of goals you can achieve. Be open to new possibilities. Not all protocols will work for you. That's okay. You'll just try the next step. Creating health is somewhat of an experiment because each of us has different genetics and our physiology changes at different points in our lives.

It's funny that we as a society believe that in order for us to be successful, we must succeed the first time at something. That is simply just a myth. If it were true, there would be no learning from failure. Yet, failure is the most effective teacher. When you were learning to walk, you fell countless times. You failed often. Did you quit? Did it occur to you that you may not ever learn? NO! You kept getting back up until you figured it out. Life is a process. It is an experience. We must go through life with the courage that we will sometimes fall or sometimes fail. But, so what! All we do is just get back up. That is the key to success. Get back up when you fall. Do not sacrifice your progress due to minor screw ups.

Phenomenal healing powers are within you waiting to be unleashed. The key is to focus on the wins, and not get distracted by the setbacks. You will get them; we all will. It is not being negative by saying this. It is being real. If you quit on yourself you will never reach your goals. Persistence regardless of setbacks is required. Nobody can heal you accept the real doctor inside, innate intelligence.

Open your heart and open your mind and begin to explore the possibility of a new life. The life I am talking about is a life with more energy, more vitality, and most of all, wellness! Become your own version of that Cali-Surfer-Perfect Life. Create your own picture of health.

Stumbling Blocks to Success

Fear can be one of the biggest obstacles that will prevent you from getting anything from this book. Fear rids you of desire and justifies why you continue to do what you do. Don't let fear hold you back. It can rob you of your dreams, and it can certainly drain you of your health and wellbeing. Perhaps our biggest fear is to be different. Different is REQUIRED to achieve health today. We have now hit a point where "normal" is the Standard American with Metabolic Disease and obesity. Even healthy kids are made fun of these days more than the fat kids because the fat kids fit in better to the norm.

Excuses will dry up your motivation more than anything out there. Don't make any more excuses. There is a saying, "It's not the situation that you are in that holds you back; it is the excuses that you use to justify the situation." Don't let excuses get in the way of you implementing what you learn from this book. Grab some strategies and go with them. See for yourself what they can do for you. Bottom line is deciding what you want, and GOING FOR IT!

Many people tell me as a doctor, "I'm tired of feeling this; I don't want to feel pain anymore." Or they may tell me, "I don't want to feel tired anymore." They tell me what they *don't* want to feel. I explain to them that if you are so concerned with what you don't want to feel, how can you concentrate on what you *do* want? So focus on what you want, not on what you don't want. That is the key! For example, if I wanted to not have knee pain, I would concentrate on increasing strength, mobility, and nutrition to the joint. I would empower my knee to heal, not just wish the pain away, complain about my luck/genetics, and expect an external force to magically fix it. There is a difference in active and passive care. You often need both to heal. For example, passive is seeing a doctor, chiropractor, massage therapist, laser, ultrasound, pain killers, etc. Active care is exercise, stretching, nutrition, mindset etc. (the majority of what this book is about.)

Technology's Role in Health Care

If you want to heal or improve, the first step is to ditch your diagnosis. Technology has had a great impact on healthcare. Our technology obsession has distracted patient care away from personal wellness and into expensive diagnostic tests. We see the evolution of the X-ray, MRI, and ultrasound that has let us see into the body what we could only approximate before. However, technology has overcomplicated health.

It gives great diagnostics but few treatments. As an example, you are not your MRI! An MRI may indicate you have a disc protrusion or a rotator cuff tear. SO WHAT? 70% of people would have a positive MRI finding whether in pain or not. Heck, I'm sure with my profession, I probably have some kind of tear in my shoulder. Does the MRI cure your protrusion or tear? No! At best these tests indicated if you are a surgical candidate or not.

The other issue with many diagnoses is that they give people an excuse not to live. People will quit exercise, work, vacation, house chores and even sex! Diagnoses can be dangerous. People will start to define themselves by their disease instead of who they really are. For example, a disc bulge is hardly ever symptomatic; you can live a pain free life with them. It often causes no dysfunction. As soon as we hear this as a diagnostic finding though, we become hesitant to live, avoiding any/all things that may stress our back. I have patients that are still afraid of a disc bulge they had in high school 30 years ago. Your body heals from spinal surgery in a few months, that disc is likely not an issue 30 years later. We get too attached to our diagnosis and assume our body is incapable of healing when that is the opposite of the truth. That 30 year old diagnosis should no longer be a problem.

This can have even more drastic effects on quality of mental health. There have been studies on how diagnoses affect patients. How it is presented makes all the difference. Whether a doctor tells a patent they will die of a disease or they tell the patient they can beat the disease, they are usually right. Suggestion is a powerful doctor. We all believe in its power. For example, one French article in Social and Science Medicine by Annememaire Jutel describes sharing a diagnosis as "dangerously transformative." There are also many cultures that believe something is incurable once they have a diagnosis. One Lebanese study showed that 7.8% of diagnosed patients believe cancer could not be cured.

Diagnoses have been a problem within the medical profession for some time. They have not brought us a higher quality of life. They only create dependent patients that believe they cannot heal or recover. The body is meant to heal. Haven't you heard of permanently paralyzed people learning to walk again? We have unlimited potential to heal once we quit believing in our detrimental prognosis. Certain individuals tend to have a superpower to achieve something after being told something is impossible. Become that person. There is no greater motivation than being told something is beyond your reach. Be courageous enough to challenge it. Do not sit back and surrender to a piece of paper or a test that told you your body was malfunctioning. Figure out how to fix the error.

I encourage you to break away from the average mentality and your diagnoses. Decide today, for yourself, that you are going to use a knowledge that will truly make a difference in your life; the innate knowledge of your physiology. It is more intelligent than any technology today. You deserve it, and those around you deserve someone who comes to the table alive, refreshed, energetic, and not just a partial representation of themselves. You deserve to reach the full you at your greatest potential! Your body is equipped with the most intense mechanisms of survival and wellbeing; we need only to unlock this potential. We need to reconstitute your genetic abilities through techniques discussed in this book.

Why do we need to think outside the box? This expression has been used for many years now and although it sounds cliché, it holds true more today than ever. We must change our paradigm from disease care, which we are clearly in, to a preventative care way of looking at health. It's the most cost effective way of taking care of our bodies. It is out of the box only because prevention is the minority of health and medicine today. Personal responsibility for our health is at an all-time low. Dependency on government, medicine, and outside forces is at an all-time high.

Prevention is not a new concept in other areas, so why should it be so under- utilized when it comes to health? The automotive companies have known about it since cars were invented. They are well aware that if you give your car preventative care such as periodic tune ups and oil changes they will last longer. It's that simple. We do not hesitate to spend $50-$1,000 on vehicle maintenance. So why do we flinch when we have to spend $40 on a copay at a doctor's office, $25 on a supplement, or even $300 on a wellness program? Do we not value ourselves and our wellbeing and performance more than our truck? Why do we do maintenance on our vehicles, but not ourselves?

The key is to invest in our fitness. Fitness is by definition the body's ability to adapt and thrive in whatever environment it is subjected to. It is not just your ability to exercise. Fitness is what we are aiming to achieve in this book. Fitness encompasses our chemical, mental and physical well-being. Be ready to take charge of your health in ways that are not covered by your health insurance. Health insurance, much like vehicle insurance, is meant for disasters and accidents. Your car insurance does not pay for oil changes right? Neither does your health insurance pay for maintenance care. Wellness is your responsibility. You need to invest in your body's oil changes, tire rotations, brakes etc. We will be discussing many types of whole body maintenance care in this book.

What Is Health?

Suppose that I were to ask you to define the term "health." What kind of answer would you give me? There is a general opinion and consensus that good health is: (1) feeling "fine," or (2) when everything is working okay, or (3) when there is an absence of pain. All of these definitions are partial and are far from complete. The World Health Organization defines health as a "state of complete physical, mental or social well-being and not merely the absence of disease or infirmity." I would argue that health is a balance of chemical, mental and physical physiology, including the body's ability to adapt to these stressors and maintain wellbeing. The body requires all three components:

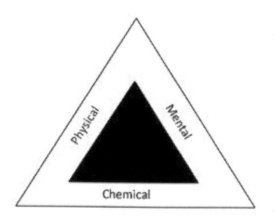

This triangle is called the triad of health. Think of a three-legged stool. Every aspect of the triangle, every leg of the chair, must be intact in order for us to stay upright. Now if health equals balance, then we can state that the opposite of health is disease, meaning a lack of balance or ease. In other words, one leg of the chair is broken. You will be seeing this triangle again. In each chapter we will be acquiring lessons to help balance one of each leg of the chair. Disease is created when an aspect of the triangle or leg on the chair is broken. Health is created, or recreated, when balance is restored.

The Withered Plant

Take a moment to think about a house plant. Let's say you came home from vacation and the leaves were dried and slumping. What would you do? I'm sure you would make sure it has water, sunlight, soil, plant food, and just overall TLC (tender loving care). Would it ever occur to you to paint the leaves green? You probably would not because the leaves would still be wilted and weak beneath that. Painting the leaves green would not fix the plant.

It's funny how common sense health can be when dealing with house plants. We do not do ourselves the same courtesy. In modern healthcare, we love to paint the leaves green. Can't make testosterone, take a hormone pill. Can't lose weight; let's put a rubber band around your stomach. You're sad, take a pill. You are in pain, another pill. Joint hurts, we will make you a new one. This is all the equivalent of painting the leaves green.

Why do we not simply look at basic needs? Much like the plant we need food, water, sun, love, etc. That is the approach we need to take towards our health. How do we stop being a withered plant? We treat the root cause, we find the deficiency, we nurture.

Painting the leaf green is the standard approach to medicine while finding the root cause is the primary concern for alternative medicine approaches. If you truly want to recreate your health and become a vibrant human like the vibrant plant on the cover, please join me on this journey. If you prefer painting the leaf green, this may not be the book for you.

Standard Medical Approach to Health

Suppose you went to your doctor for a mild symptom? Maybe you have headaches. Maybe you have bad menstrual cramps, pain in your feet, knee pain, arthritis, fever, or muscle spasms. Would your common physician not just tell you to take some Ibuprofen and be on your way?

How would you react to a mechanic that told you that all you need to do for your car is bring it in and have the oil changed when the car starts to give you problems? Is an oil change the fix for every car trouble incident? No? Usually further diagnostics are required and specific fixes must be implemented to different parts of the car. It is similar with the body; Ibuprofen should not be used to fix each and every dysfunction. It is not a cure all, it is a cover up, numbing your brain to what your body is screaming for you to listen to. Period cramps, headaches and foot pain are not the body's deficiency in ibuprofen just like all car trouble is not a deficiency in oil. They are a red flag similar to your check engine light. The body can have a deficiency in omega 3's which makes us desire more ibuprofen. Omega 3 is like the oil in the vehicle. We know what the consequences of not getting maintenance checks and oil changes in our car, which incidentally we will only have for 10 years at best. Yet we don't always give our bodies(that we will hopefully have for many decades), the same kind of preventative care.

Do not ignore your bodies check engine lights and red flags. Do not cover them up with ibuprofen and then act surprised when more severe health problems arise.

The Magic Pill Lifestyle

Why do we put so little effort into maintaining our bodies? That is because most people believe that there is a magic pill that will solve all of our problems. That is why we often ignore our body's check engine light, we think emergency medicine will save us. Emergency medicine is amazing in this country, and they are exhausted with the overflow of avoidable health disparities.

The birth of modern medicine could be attributed to the time when Robert Koch postulated the germ theory in 1860. Once this discovery took place, it was emphasized and widely believed that microbes were the cause of ALL disease. It was also widely accepted that the key to health was to destroy those foreign enemies with antibiotics and antibacterial drugs. They eliminated the option of bodily dysfunction due to the environment we put it in, and instead became obsessed with creating a pill for everything while ignoring the root cause. We all recognize that cancer for example may be due to toxins in our home or workplace. My grandfather died due to toxins on the ship he worked on in the army for example. This was not due to a bug, it was due to the environment. Your body's also influenced by other factors. These generally fall under categories: thoughts, traumas and toxins. The environment created inside your body or the external environment you are in daily plays the biggest role in your overall health. The biggest influence is not always an infection. The fix for everything is not a pill; it is addressing the root cause of the dysfunction. It is addressing the chemical, mental, and emotional factors involved in the internal and external environment.

The germ theory has resulted in the overuse of antibiotics to the point that we are now dealing with super-strains of bacteria and viruses. These microbes are becoming more and more resistant to all of the antibiotics originally created to fight them off. We put antibiotics in all our food, prescribe it for every sniffly nose, and use it preventatively for every surgery, even getting a tooth pulled. It's gone too far. There are many more factors to health than bugs. The five main factors are: food, toxins, bugs, traumas and hormones. Most of these factors have become overwhelming in today's society and this book will give you tools as a defense against the confusion.

Alternative Health Options

People today are becoming more and more aware of alternatives. They are sick and tired of being sick and tired and they want options. They want to know why they are sick or why they are feeling a certain way, not just another ibuprofen, steroid or antibiotic. They are sick and tired of hearing obscure explanations on what they have and why taking a "magic pill" will solve all their problems.

We are getting smarter. In the United States, in the year 2001 there were more visits to Alternative Health Care practitioners than traditional allopathic medical doctors. It may have started with the baby boomers who wanted to create and maintain health, not just mask their problems with drugs and surgery. We are not being attacked by the flu. We are not innocent victims being chosen by microbes. We are in fact creating the very environment for these bacteria and viruses to feast upon a body that is full of toxicity. You can't just blame the doctors here either. It is the responsibility of each individual to care for themselves and to take action to prevent disease. Your doctor did not force feed you junk and glue you to the sofa. Your couch and carbohydrate disease is all on you.

Health Insanity

Anyone can change their attitude and approach to health, but if you continue to look at your body the same way you have in the past, you will continue to get what you have gotten in the past. "The definition of insanity is doing the same thing over and over and expecting different results." – A. Einstein. Quit being an insane person, if you want to change things, start with your mindset. You must stop looking at your body as a piece of dysfunctional equipment and recognize it for the ultimate intelligence it actually possesses. You must prioritize your health, not as something that should be tolerated, but something that must be maintained and even improved.

In life, it seems we only do consistently that which we find important enough to make a priority. It is important, therefore, to look at your health as something that is so important that it becomes top priority. We always find it comical that people will spend $50 on a bottle of booze, a haircut, a nice dinner, or a pair of jeans but will complain about spending this with a doctor or on a supplement. You must change your mindset and invest in your health instead of only spending money on items intended to be luxuries. We have had patients turn down care in our office due to cost and then drive off in a Cadillac or we see them at the Kroger across the street buying booze and cigarettes. Start to realize expenses related to your survival and you will likely find ample funds to create health. As an example in my life, Crossfit is an expensive sport. When I found it, my gym charged $80-$120 a month! I thought there was no way I could maintain that. So I changed my mind set. I said, instead of spending $40-$100 on bars and restaurants each weekend, I would buy a membership. I would invest in my health, instead of destroying it with alcohol.

Starting Your Way Back to Health

Start to ask yourself, "What can I do today to start on a path of wellness?" I recommend that my patients make the changes that are very easy to do. For example, I had a patient who had not exercised in many, many years. I asked her if she could spend 5 minutes a day just stretching. Of course that sounded very easy to do. Before long, that 5 minute stretch turned into 10 minutes. Next, she realized that the stretching really felt good and added some light resistance to her routine with some hand weights. By the end of a month, she had added cardiovascular exercise to the routine and was up to a half hour of exercising. It felt so good that the habit was one she intended on maintaining. This book is structured around these types of recommendations.

You see once you create a habit, you can expand upon it, but you will set yourself up for failure if you start too big. The most important thing that I want you to get out of this chapter is the subtle consequences our choices have on our health. There are small decisions we make every day that can make the difference between being completely well or not. Conversely, you don't have to jump into being a complete health nut in 30 days. There are certain folks that have a cult like approach to health and fitness, that level of dedication is not required. In fact, I will say there is such a thing as being too "healthy." The paradox in this is that some individuals become so obsessed with health that they forget to live, and this produces its own set of consequences. The thing to remember with this is that health will look different to everyone. Do not strive to be someone you are not, but be healthy according to your quality of life standards. Not everyone is training to climb Everest, am I right?

This book is aimed to help you define your health, attain it, and sustain it.

There will be 12 steps, or 12 months of new challenges to find and maintain long term health. Each step will address a chemical, mental, and physical component of health in congruence with the triad of health. These steps can help you eliminate a disease creating physiology as well as become the Fit-Cali-Perfect Surfer, or your own interpretation of true health.

It is important to remember, as I said before, new goals must always be set and strived for. Quitting after 1 year will likely not get you there. We are in this for the long haul. We want long term, gradual, and positive change. I know my health journey has been life-long, I am not where I want to be but I am so much farther when I started about 8 years ago. I will be presenting this book in a journey similar to my own.

My Journey

I will be honest; I grew up in a fairly healthy household. I thought we were the biggest health freaks growing up. We bought organic food, my mom took us to Alternative Medicine doctors, we exercised and traveled as a family, played sports, had salads packed in our lunch, etc. I have been used to being food shamed since eating tuna for lunch in elementary school. So I cannot say I am from a background with no foundation for lifestyle changes. I was always the fitness freak on my sports teams and my coaches often joked about me having to do push-ups on the bus to softball games because I was that obsessed. My nickname was "Beast" or "Guns" due to my workout habits. I was one of only a few girls in weights class at the time. I won't say I was 100% healthy though despite my habits. I had morning nausea all through high school. I never felt great until at least 3rd hour. I also was taken to the doctor for abdominal pain more than once. There was no definitive diagnosis, just a suspicion for ovarian cysts. I had severe seasonal allergies and depended on Claritin. I was also very much into the energy drink scene.

I cannot give you an epic I lost 100 pounds and changed my life kind of story. However, I will tell you the secret to my success, I ALWAYS found new goals and pushed toward them. Anytime I stood still and tried to simply maintain, I would slowly slip out of shape, gain weight, get inflamed, get joint pain, etc.

It wasn't until partway through college that I realized, there were more ways of chasing optimal health than just generalized diet, weight loss, and exercise. It happened when I traveled to Australia for a summer while attending the University of Michigan. I was a bit healthier than most college students. I cooked my own meals, went jogging, lifted weights, but I still partied a lot, binge watched Netflix, and reaped the consequences. The combo of travel and undergrad lifestyle left me with extreme gut issues. I had not had a normal bowel movement for an entire summer before I sought help. I had stool tests that all came back negative. I was very frustrated that I was so uncomfortable. I was afraid to run to far from my house for fear of an accident. I knew where the bathroom was at every store. Thankfully, my mom took me for food allergy testing. I ranked extremely high for dairy. I went all in and took all dairy out of my life, which I realized then had been about ¾ of my diet. I was finally able to hold my bowels and actually lost some weight in the process. I consider this the real beginning to my wellness revolution. I started to see how what I ate truly affected my overall wellbeing.

Fast forward to graduate school at Logan College of Chiropractic. I still had some bowel issues even post-dairy-free changes. I occasionally suffered the lower abdominal pain of high school and was stuck home in bed with it about twice a year. During Chiropractic school, I started getting adjusted regularly. We were assigned to an upper-classmen that would doctor us. One day I noticed, I had not purchased Claritin in months. My allergies had become near non-existent. I never suffered much from back pain or other stereotypical chiropractic care conditions so I was amazed by this seemingly unrelated observation. Soon I joined a business management chiropractic group called Maximized Living. It was there that I learned about all the health advancement chiropractic had to offer. This group incorporated nutrition, adjustments, mindset, detox, and fitness into one package. Through this I discovered Crossfit from my friend Liz. Crossfit changed me more than any health program up to that point. It taught me about the importance of group exercise, accountability, high intensity interval training, and The Paleo Diet. Now I am the "all in" personality, so naturally I went into Paleo lifestyle quickly. I felt better than I had before in my life! The energy, the toned muscles, the fun community, I loved it all. Only problem was, I was still having that dang abdominal pain.

I believe things are presented to you when you need them the most. That is when I met Dr. Scott Huff. He was a local Chiropractor that did MORE! He did Functional Medicine, Applied Kinesiology, blood work, allergy tests, genetics tests, biomechanics coaching and above all, taught you about true health. I was really struggling to figure out how I wanted to practice chiropractic. As soon as my sister and I had our first appointment, there was no question in my mind that this was what I wanted to do and how I wanted to do it. As an added bonus, he fixed my abdominal pain visit #1! He also gave me the tools to prevent its onset in the future. Through this doctor, I went through leaky gut protocols, detox protocols, changed my biomechanics and adjusted my whole philosophy on health. My athletic performance skyrocketed, I reached 20 lbs. increase in personal records within a month.

I was most of the way through my doctorate at this point and was ready to take on a whole new skill set and education. I threw myself into his teachings and his mentors. After learning a great deal from the Applied Kinesiology Research Center, Functional Medicine teachings of Dr. Kharrazian and earning my Masters in Nutrition, Dr. Huff took me under his wing. I was able to practice and train with him for a year. Upon the graduation of my husband, Dr. Travis Tourjee, we wanted to move closer to family. This is when we landed our practice in Port Huron, MI.

Together, Dr. Travis and I continued to reach for more. We pushed ourselves athletically, mentally and nutritionally every day. We still do Crossfit together, it is how we met. See what I mean about health and fitness affecting more than just your waistline? We both experiment with different nutritional protocols including Keto, intermittent fasting, gut repair etc. Lastly, we have made an effort to include other alternative medicine technicians into our wellness team. We get regular massages, see an acupuncturist, and talk to health coaches; each provides us with different benefits. Finding a healthcare team is another thing we will discuss in this book. So, let's get started!

Month 1

Chiropractic, Optimal Digestion, and Journaling

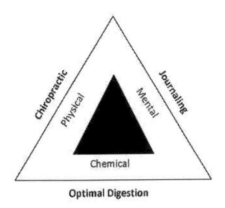

Optimal Digestion

My Experience

The number of things chiropractic has helped me with is astounding. I never cease to be amazed. There are times in my life I have struggled with terrible stomach pain, lower abdominal pain, dizziness, IBS, or just regular muscle/joint pain that were not managed with any lifestyle changes. When my stomach acts up, diet changes just are not enough to relieve it; at least not in a timely fashion. Chiropractic got rid of my hospitalizing lower abdominal pain.

I am pretty hard on my body, between my profession and my exercise, adjustments to my spine and other joints literally keep me employed and functioning. The main way that I track my health changes and improvements is through journaling. Through all protocols listed in this book, I was also receiving chiropractic care. I tracked my progress and the speed of recovery. I can tell you with absolute certainty that my patients trying to do diet and lifestyle changes alone do not recover as quickly. Every time I have a nutrition only patient, chiropractic care always takes their care to a higher efficiency.

Chiropractic

I know it is somewhat selfish to mention my profession first but let me take a moment to defend myself. It takes a lot of motivation to start any health journey. Having pain, or other dysfunctional physiology, makes it very difficult to even start. We will go into pain mechanisms in depth later, but in short, pain changes you. It destroys your brain. It exhausts you. It can make you angry, impulsive, and unlike yourself. Finding a chiropractor before many other steps will help you get your bodily processes optimized before you make any extreme changes. Often you will find that some problems are cleared up from chiropractic care alone as I did with my seasonal allergies. Your first assignment is to find a chiropractor. If you do not connect with the first one, keep searching. Each practitioner is different.

I think chiropractic can span all three categories of the triad of health. We act as personal counselors, nutrition coaches, and exercise enthusiasts. We help people with every element. Our biggest influence however, is on the physical; the structure of the nervous system and its integration with every cell tissue and organ in our body. We are one of the few professions that try to optimize primal physiology. We believe in the body's ability to heal: innate intelligence. We believe that if there is an interference with innate intelligence, the system is subluxated. Subluxations must be removed to allow the body to heal at its full potential. Subluxations are any disconnect between mind and body, usually addressed as a bone out of place in simple terms.

Subluxations may be of mental, chemical, or physical origin. Physically, you may have a bone, organ, muscle, or joint that requires correction. You may need to exercise more, stretch, or rest. Chemically, you may need a specific nutrient, detoxification, or environmental change. Mentally, you may need less stress, better relationships, more family time, or the consult of professionals.

I always get the question "Doc, why do things come out of place?" The answer is within any aspect of the triad of health. That is why it is the focus of this book.

Hands-on Healing

Chiropractic is also a very powerful healing technique because it is hands-on. Many health care disciplines do not use hands-on approach with their patients, with some exceptions like massage, acupuncture, and physical therapy. Physical touch has some healing attributes on its own. Think about a mother's touch when you are sick. Her rubbing your back when you were ill always added comfort and relieved some distress.

Healing techniques like this allow the practitioner to feel where there are imbalances in the structure in order to correct them. Whether a bone is out of place, a muscle is strained, an acupuncture point is knotted, or a joint is off kilter; physical touch is the one diagnostic procedure that will identify them.

If there is any kind of interference within or surrounding the nervous system it causes dis-ease or creates a situation where you are not completely well. Often that interference can't be felt by the patient, only the practitioner. There may be no pain or pressure at all to tell you something isn't right. A doctor that utilizes their hands on your tissue will be able to identify maladies before the patient has severe symptoms.

Our Education

The reason we can coach patients on so many aspects of health lies within our education. Chiropractic is a doctorate degree. Most students earn their Bachelors of Science first. I have my Bachelor's of Microbiology from the University of Michigan. Our graduate program requires a curriculum close to medical school's. We take classes in chiropractic techniques, biochemistry, nutrition, obstetrics, dermatology, anatomy, physiology, pediatrics, business, etc. Most schools also offer congruent master's programs. I earned my Master's in Nutrition while in Chiropractic School. We have 4,620 hours of classroom education, very comparable to the medical doctor's 4,800. Our education prepares us to be the optimal gateway physician: we connect all health complaints, treat the nervous system, and make specific further health recommendations or referrals.

How Chiropractic Works

Our body is a series of circuits linked together to form the nervous system. The circuit goes from the brain, down an afferent nerve to a muscle, organ, or tissue and back up to the brain via the efferent nerve. Chiropractic plays a vital role in allowing this loop, our innate intelligence, to do its job. When subluxations occur, those blockages reduce the messages transmitted by the nerve, then the body's ability to correct what might be wrong is hindered. Regular, preventative chiropractic care is what will allow a free flow of signals to all areas of the body.

A unique chiropractic technique that truly enhances this loop is Applied Kinesiology. Applied Kinesiology (AK) is one of many chiropractic techniques. Did you know that all chiropractors practice somewhat differently? That is because we are offered at least 15 techniques per school to choose from. The value in multiple techniques is that different methods work better for certain patients. For example, Webster technique is used specifically for pregnancy. Logan Basic technique is a gentle one used for children. There really is something for everyone.

What makes AK so useful is that it incorporates the triad of health in each and every treatment. It is a diagnostic technique that allows the doctor to identify the main areas of dysfunction and focus their efforts on treating that instead of all the secondary symptoms.

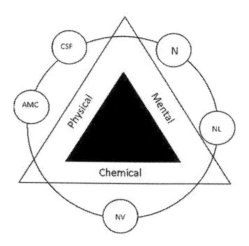

NL=Neurolymphatic
AMC=Acupuncture Meridian
NV=Neurovascular
CSF=Cerebrospinal Fluid
N=Nerve

Applied Kinesiology incorporates many systems into its approach. As shown in the photo above, it incorporates nerve, neuro-vascular, cerebrospinal fluid, acupuncture meridian, and neuro-lymphatic relationships into treatments. This is in addition to the triad of health we spoke about earlier. AK also incorporates muscle-organ interactions. For example, muscle contraction in the abdominal wall, muscles such as Quadratus Lumborum, are vital to optimal digestion. All patients with digestive dysfunction will have one or many muscles around the abdominal cavity that are not engaging properly. These muscles are required to create internal pressure to keep the bowels moving. There are many of these relationships throughout the body with muscles and organs. Our musculoskeletal system is tightly integrated with other internal systems.

A typical treatment with an AK practitioner should go something like this:

1. Posture Evaluation to look for muscular imbalance.

2. Test for muscle contraction and hold in areas of suspected dysfunction

3. Evaluate for triad of health or 5 factors above that may be related to dysfunction in the muscle. This is done through certain reflex points and nutrients.

4. Identification of neurological factors or subluxations involved in the dysfunction

5. Correction of neurology, specific muscle treatments, often cranial work

6. Lifestyle recommendations to prevent further dysfunction in the area.

The Spine and Gut Connection

Hippocrates was a healer well before his time. My favorite three quotes from him are:

"All disease begins in the gut."

"Let food be thy medicine and thy medicine be thy food."

"Look well to the spine for the cause of disease."

He was far ahead of western medicine in these thoughts; we are now just beginning to realize how right he was. There are at least two nervous systems in the body. One is housed in the spine, the other in your gut.

While each is communicating with the other through nerves and chemicals, they each may require their own treatments.

The gut houses the majority of your immune system. That is because it is your most vulnerable site to the outside world. We are constantly inoculating it with whatever we put in our mouths. Think of how many things per day touch your lips or nostrils, and then you swallow whatever enters your nose or mouth, which goes to the stomach. Once germs get to the stomach, most infectious material is neutralized by the stomach acid, if it makes it past this (for reasons we will discuss) the immune cells of the gut should take care of it or your other digestive enzymes. However, in today's society there are many interruptions with the gut lining, stomach acid, and digestive enzymes. Therefore, many foreign proteins get into our body that shouldn't and wreak havoc. It is important to optimize digestion. Both of your nervous systems are your master controllers to the body.

Healthy Digestion

When it comes to digestion, not a single person will have the same optimal diet as another. <u>Your connection with food is very personal</u>. What jives well with your body can be determined by genetics, fetal nutrition, previous sickness, mental stress, or how your food is grown. Therefore, learning what to and what not to incorporate in your diet is highly experimental. Food diaries are not to be underestimated. Not every intolerance, allergy, or sensitivity can be detected on a lab test. The best doctor is the one inside of you. Remember innate intelligence? You know better than anyone else what your body is telling you. So don't let social media and popular beliefs make you have a miserable belly each day. As a general rule it is best to stick to 5 food groups: meat, vegetable, fruit, sweet potato, or coconut. But this book will delve into many specific diets for certain conditions and help you find your perfect food lifestyle. The first assignment will be simply to eliminate known food triggers that create reactions in YOUR body. Before we can discuss elimination requirements though, it is important to understand normal digestion.

Normal Digestion Progression

Step 1 - Ideally, ingested food is first broken down by chewing and enzymes in the mouth called amylase. This is the first area that can be inadequate. Many people scarf down meals without enough chewing and hence not enough enzyme activity. This overburdens the stomach and can cause inadequate food breakdown and lead to heartburn or undigested food getting to the gut which feeds bad bacteria.

Step 2 - The stomach acid, HCL (hydrochloric acid), aids in protein breakdown and vitamin/mineral absorption. However, many are on proton pump inhibitors like prilosec or a strong base like TUMS which destroys stomach acid. This can lead to more undigested food feeding bad bacteria as well as conditions like anemia or protein/mineral/vitamin deficiencies. This also complicates heartburn. Most people get heartburn due to increased acid production, but not from normal stomach acid. In most cases of heartburn, undigested food sits around and rots. The putrefying food produces an acid that causes heartburn symptoms. This acid is neutralized by tums or similar products. This makes people feel great but does not fix the problem or the ensuing deficiencies. To aid this step, we often need to slow down our eating, take digestive enzymes or zinc, or massage the stomach.

Step 3 - Enzymes from the pancreas further digest protein and carbohydrates. A sluggish pancreas from constant stress and fluctuating blood sugar can inhibit the ability to fully digest these particles and again lead to undigested food in the gut to feed bad bacteria. In this particular area of digestion, the primary outcome is SIBO, small intestinal bacterial overgrowth or leaky gut. (Chapter 6)

Step 4 - Bile from the gallbladder emulsifies fat for digestion. This can be interrupted from liver toxicity. The liver produces bile and can be slowed down by excess hormones, heavy metals, blood sugar instability, birth control, bowel toxicity and more. If you are unable to properly digest fats, the result will be a deficiency leading to hormone deregulation and brain dysfunction. (Chapter 7)

Step 5 - The gut wall of intestine absorbs nutrients. These nutrients go to veins and then to the liver. The liver filters the blood before it can go to the body. This is another area where the liver may get overwhelmed. If there are excess toxins in the food, an infection in the gut, Leaky gut lining letting food particles into the blood, or prescription medication harming the lining can devastate this system. (Chapter 10)

Step 6 - After the liver filters the blood and makes the necessary modifications to it, the blood flows to the heart and then the rest of the body.

Step 7 - Elimination of waste. You should have a bowel movement every day. You should excrete the length of your forearm and diameter of your index finger to thumb circled. Otherwise you are gaining toxicity from your own waste. Many patients get relief from GI complaints by getting a chiropractic adjustment. Reconnecting the brain with the body can cause significant change especially with constipation. Therefore, on top of any diet or lifestyle changes recommend in this book, I suggest you get adjusted. You will usually see sub-optimal change without chiropractic care.

Food Reactions

Many people associate food reactions with allergies. However, this is not the only mechanism behind bad food effects. Depending on an allergy test to explain symptoms will leave the majority of patients misdiagnosed and miserable. Before we delve into the many diets to help with poor food reactions I want to delineate the mechanisms we will discuss. The three main reactions can be described as intolerance, sensitivity, or allergy.

Intolerance: If you eat these it will cause serious damage.

If you have these reactions, the correlated food MUST be avoided including small contaminations from food preparation. You either lack the enzymes to digest the food, or the body attacks it with severe consequences. For example, if you are lactose intolerant, it is not an allergy. You lack the enzyme to break down the lactose protein which produces symptoms when the body reacts to the undigested protein. If the body has such an immune reaction to the food that the products destroy your own tissue, or trickily target your immune cells against your own body, you have a problem. This is what happens in cases such as Celiac or Hashimoto's disease. The body sees gluten, attacks it, the attack cells are blind pac-men for the most part so they attack any tissue that looks like the gluten protein, in this case the gut lining and thyroid. Gut lining destruction leads to Celiac Disease and thyroid destruction leads to Hashimoto's.

Allergy: produces a histamine response or antibodies (IgE, IgG, or IgA)

When giving up a food to see if it is causing allergies, you must eliminate it 100%. Even a thumb sized portion can destroy your progress depending on sensitivity. The only way to know if a food is increasing your allergies is to give it up completely and then bring it back a few weeks later and see what it does to you. Allergy symptoms are not always what you think. Only anaphylactic (Epi pen worthy) allergies produce a typical response. There are two types of allergic responses: delayed and immediate.

Delayed- A few hours to a few days after you consume a food you may get a "stomach migraine" or other digestive symptoms all the way to acne breakouts. A full list of allergy symptoms is listed below. The point here is that it takes the immune system a few days to make these antibodies and react. These are driven by IgG antibodies. IgG is a number you may see on allergy tests.

Allergy Symptoms

Acne	Recurring Infection
Eczema	Auto-immune disease
Sinusitis	Insomnia
Gas	ADD
Bloating	Headache
Diarrhea	Weight gain
Fatigue	Hypoglycemia
Joint pain	Cysts
Asthma	

Immediate- This is how we typically attribute allergies. You drink milk and your nose stuffs up and your throat gets phlegmy. Worst case scenario, it can lead to anaphylactic shock. This is typically an IgE or histamine response. IgE and IgG are separate immune signal cells.

Sensitivity: you have a reaction, non-specific, unknown why, difficult to diagnose. Food sensitivities may cause fatigue, gas, bloating, mood swings, nervousness, migraines and eating disorders. Testing for these is very tedious. Sensitivity can be caused by many mechanisms. It may be from a poor bacterial balance in the gut, a psychological association, or inability to handle toxicity.

As a general rule, if you react to a food poorly, quit eating it. It may be an allergy, sensitivity, or intolerance. Regardless of the definition, that food is not beneficial, it is harmful to your system.

Some sensitivity is due to the actual consistency or fiber content of a food. For example, certain foods will aggravate your narrow gut valves. A common example we see regularly as AK chiropractors is Ileocecal Valve Syndrome (ICV).

Ileocecal Valve Syndrome

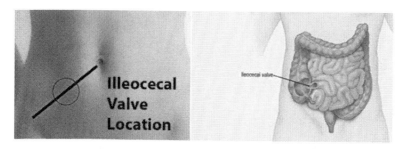

www.triadofhealth.net

As you can see in the photos, the Ileocecal Valve is a structure located in the lower right quadrant of the abdomen. Its purpose is to prevent backflow of material from the large to small intestine. It also prevents bacteria (which is abundant in the large intestine), from flowing into the small intestine (where there is little bacteria).

When the ICV becomes a symptomatic (painful) problem is when it becomes stuck open, stuck closed, or is constantly irritated by offending foods. This problem can be relieved by your Applied Kinesiology doctor, however, if the offending foods are not eliminated the problem is likely to return.

This problem typically presents as lower abdominal pain in the location pictured. It may feel like a muscle cramp, present pain during sex, hurt when using the restroom, or simply be tender to touch. Though you may have no symptoms at all! I have seen it refer pain all the way to shoulders and knees. If you have an unrelenting pain problem that gets worse after holidays or any other time you binge on the listed offending foods, it may be ICV related. I can say from personal experience, when I get pain in my right knee, eliminating ICV inflammation will clear up my knee pain.

If you have lower abdominal pain in this area that is severe or accompanied by a fever, please seek help immediately. You may be suffering appendix pain. I went to the hospital for this exact pain, thinking it was my appendix. This was the condition my chiropractor addressed with me to fix my abdominal pain episodes.

To aid ICV at home, I recommend pressure and cold packs to the area. You or your partner may hold down on the area for minutes at a time, this may "reset" the valve. However, it is usually not this simple so I recommend seeing an Applied Kinesiology Chiropractor who can neurologically fix it and aid you with proper supplements. Bile salts or chlorophyll can help this condition. I would also recommend avoiding the offending foods listed here.

Offending foods

- Bread
- Caffeine
- Spicy
- Sugary
- Nuts/Seeds
- Roughage
- Popcorn
- Alcohol
- Junk Food
- Corn
- Milk
- Wheat
- Soy
- Parasites
- Unhealthy oils
- legumes

Now that you are familiar with different reactions, you should be able to indicate a few foods from this list to start your elimination program. With this increased knowledge, you also may start to notice symptoms and food that bother you that had been previously ignored or attributed to other things. The best way to track your gut symptoms through this phase will be with a food diary.

Schedules and Journals

The absolute best way to keep accountable with your journey is to document it. This is especially true with tracking for food reactions. Remember, delayed type reactions can take 4 or more days to manifest. It is important to have a journal saying what you ate. Most people cannot remember what they had for dinner last night, let alone an allergy exposure form a week ago.

Some of us are better with technology while others like handwritten notes. I am terrible at phone tracking with food apps and such. The most effective way I found to track progress was to get an old fashioned planner/journal; basically a planner with a lot of extra writing space per day. This helped for many reasons:

1. I scheduled workout times

2. I tracked my food. If I had a bad health day, I could look back over the previous week and find a cause. If I didn't lose weight I could easily see how many cheat meals I had etc.

3. It kept me accountable by being able to always look back at my details.

4. I tracked my weight and measurements month by month. I keep these planners and can look back even a few years to see where I was at.

5. I tracked symptoms every day. I tracked sleep, digestion, energy, acne, menstrual cycles, or any other oddities.

6. I was more organized and productive with a scheduler.

7. I decreased stress by having my days, weeks, months organized in front of me.

8. I set new goals each month and keep them in my visual. These were categorized as physical or mental. You may want to eat better, so be specific and list the types of foods you will avoid to obtain better health. If you want to learn a new skill or improve a relationship, list specific actions you can take. The more specific you are with goals the more successful you will be.

A useful stress reduction technique that leads to increased productivity is routine. I recommend setting one and making it visual, whether on the wall in the kitchen or in your journal. Some of the most successful individuals schedule their day from sun up to sun down. They schedule play time, family time, work time, exercise time etc. So I challenge you to find, implement, and stick to your routine. I find it works best when you have things the same time a day throughout the week/month. For example, we do 6 AM Crossfit. That is my workout time. Wednesday nights are family dinner. Sunday evenings are movie lazy time. Friday afternoons are for house projects. That way your body gets accustomed to doing certain activities on certain days/times. If you miss this schedule you will feel guilty or you will feel like something is missing. That is good, it keeps you accountable. We are like kids, we do better with routine.

This month's assignments:

Start a planner, food counter, exercise tracker, etc.

Find a chiropractor

Eliminate Known/Suspected food triggers in order to optimize digestion

Month 2

Inflammation, Movement, and Being Social

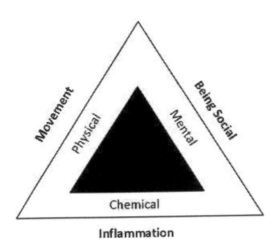

My Experience

I am not sure when it started, but at some point over the past few years I started experiencing knee pain. I have not had any imaging done but I would be willing to bet there is something wrong with my meniscus. I will tell you I had it adjusted, I had acupuncture, laser therapy, and massage therapy. None of these worked. How frustrating right? I address these issues for a living.

So, I had to take a step back for a moment and try to figure out why this was happening. I had no initial injury, no muscle strain. I do yoga. I lift weights. I do all the right things to have a mechanically sound knee, save for possibly squatting too heavy at times. The one thing I could figure about my knee, was that it was chronically inflamed from diet and stress. I figured out the pain didn't start from the gym, it started after grad school when I was starting a business, building a practice, getting married, living at home, and basically having no filter on my diet. I had been eating more grains than usual. I was drinking more days that I should have. I was not meal prepping. I was eating out more. The 2012 version of me would have been thoroughly disgusted. I had gotten busy, had a few huge life changes thrown at me and started to make excuses. I forgot, or blocked out, how much my diet affected me. Finally, I said "Enough!"

I got back on track. I went drastic and cut out carbohydrates almost completely for a month followed by a 6 week gut repair and liver cleanse. In the first two weeks I noticed my knee pain was almost gone. I now recognize that as soon as I get too carb crazy, or drink too much, or over-caffeinate and under eat that the pain slowly creeps back. I have to keep my inflammation under control. I also recognize that if my knee hurts from inflammation, there are likely other body processes that suffer as well. I can say menstrual cramps go right along with it as an example.

Inflammation can be a hard thing to control depending on your lifestyle. If you are a type A, workaholic, coffee drinking, heavy lifting person it can be a delicate balance to stay on top of it all. If you are a yoga master, dialed in diet, get enough sleep, and control your workload kind of person then you may heal faster and keep inflammation in check easier. You have to remember, chronic stress is inflammatory. Your stress load directly affects how easy or hard it is to keep your pain under control. This is where it gets tricky for me, as a physician, to treat some patients. Things like family health stress throw your system for such a loop that adjustments alone will not heal you all the way. The stress must be addressed as well. That is the only way to decrease the inflammation enough to heal. So what exactly is this inflammation that causes so much trouble? What contributes to it? How do we control it? Let's discuss this process.

Inflammation

Inflammation is at the center of most modern diseases. As such, it will be the focus of many protocols included in these chapters. We will begin by defining the inflammation epidemic and discussing how to battle it with an anti-inflammatory diet and lifestyle.

Inflammation is a normal immune reaction triggered by a perceived attack on our body from bacteria or trauma. Inflammation creates redness, heat, swelling, pain and eventually loss of function. In order to create this cascade, we use pain creation molecules such as prostaglandins, corticosteroids, cytokines, and lymphocytes. These are the target of most anti-inflammatory medications. For example, ibuprofen targets the prostaglandins and steroids mimic corticosteroids. However, there are ways to modulate these cells with changes in nutrition. For example, the omega 3's in fish oil changes prostaglandin production similar to ibuprofen. This can decrease pain and the overall inflammatory reaction.

Our body creates inflammatory molecules to protect our cells from infection but by chronically stimulating this mechanism we are killing ourselves. Therefore, the key is to stop creating this cascade. You should be using your body's innate inflammatory reactions for infection and disease. You should not be constantly barraging it with poor lifestyle choices. We constantly stimulate this reaction through 5 factors.

The 5 causes of Inflammation are:

Food - pesticides, additives, coloring, man-made food like products, sugar

Trauma/Stress - physical injury or emotional stress

Toxins - air/water quality, work environment, our liver's ability to eliminate waste

Bugs - any infection of bacteria, yeast, fungus, or parasite

Hormones - in our food, medications, water and insulin resistance

It is reasonable to claim that over 90% of disease in America are due to these factors and the chronic inflammation they cause. To give you a better visual, take your five fingernails and start to itch the back of your other hand. After a few moments this will become uncomfortable. You will experience the redness, swelling, heat and pain portions of inflammation. After less than a day you would likely have gone through the skin and caused a full loss in skin function in that area. With the same experiment I could say take 4 fingers away but keep going with only your index finger. The redness, swelling, heat, pain and loss of function would still happen right? That is what happens when you fix 4/5 of the factors. Let's say you change your diet, detox, decrease stress, kill all the bad bugs BUT you stay on birth control. The birth control hormone would be the index finger still scratching away ruining your skin. I hope this helps you understand that often all five factors must be addressed to get inflammation under control. We will address all 5 throughout the book. Without any substantial changes to our diet and lifestyle patterns, people will keep on suffering from inflammatory diseases. For a complete list of inflammation causes and solutions, see the appendix.

Inflammation Disorders

There are various health issues connected with inflammation. Some of the most commonly seen are numerous kinds of arthritis. Arthritis is a broad term that refers to various kinds of inflammation in the joint area. Some of the most frequent/common kinds of inflammation-triggered arthritis are:

- Rheumatoid arthritis
- Degenerative Arthritis
- Bursitis
- Tendinitis
- Fibromyalgia
- Joint Pain
- Osteoarthritis

Unfortunately, inflammation is not just about pain. It is also an underlying cause for metabolic diseases such as heart disease, cancer, diabetes, Alzheimer's, and obesity.

Shockingly enough, the World Health Organization reveals that over 13 million people annually lose their lives from cardiovascular disorders. The cancer rates are also alarmingly high, with 8 million people losing their lives from cancer annually. Both of these dangerous disorders are caused by chronic inflammation. So, in order to control the likelihood of developing such disorders, we must adopt some healthier diet and lifestyle changes.

To give an example, this is how the inflammatory cascade can lead to heart disease:

1. Insulin is released due to increased blood sugar from carbohydrate meal (pasta, fries, etc.)

2. Insulin is extremely inflammatory when chronically induced and becomes unchecked in the system (Diabetes)

3. Inflammatory chemicals create artery micro-tears because they damage out healthy cells

4. The body uses cholesterol in attempts to patch the torn artery

5. Chronic use of cholesterol forms a plaque

6. The plaque narrows the artery which decreases blood flow, changes blood pressure, and leads to stroke when the plaque is detached

Inflammatory Food

For those affected by inflammation, diets rich in carbs and low in protein intake can be destructive while the opposite diet (low carb/high protein intake), actually keeps inflammation under control and all the negative side effects connected to it.

Every individual organism differs from the other, and thus it is important to spot all the signs and symptoms we experience when we take certain foods. The symptom list is numerous as we discussed in the previous chapter. I will offer you many nutrition regimens against inflammation later in this book, but at this point, let's delve into a few basics.

Some of the foods that trigger an inflammatory response in the body are:

1: Sugar/Sweets. High amounts of sugar consumption have been associated with weight issues, inflammation, and chronic inflammatory diseases like Diabetes Mellitus. Processed sugars and foods with an elevated Glycemic Index (G.I), raise insulin levels and trigger an immune system response.

2: Typical vegetable oils for cooking and baking. Oils with a high omega-6 fatty acid/low omega-3 acid ratio, also lead to inflammation. These include canola oil, sunflower, safflower, vegetable, shortening, Crisco, and peanut oil/butter. Yes, peanut butter is extremely inflammatory and creates bad pain cascades. I know it stinks but it is something to consider if you finish a container a week.

3: Trans fats. These fats are typically found in junk food/fast food meals. Not only are they associated with inflammation, but also insulin resistance and other chronic disorders.

4: Non-organic milk and dairy products. Non-organic dairy products can also result in inflammation, especially in the female population, due to the hormones and allergen attributes they contain.

5: Conventional red or processed meat. Eating red and processed meat is also associated with immune reactions that lead to chronic inflammation within our systems.

Other types of foods suspected of causing inflammation are grains/flour, alcohol, synthetic food preservatives, and grain-fed meats. All the above foods should be avoided if any signs of inflammation emerge.

For the purpose of this chapter I would like you to focus on eliminating the No 1-5 foods. We will gradually get through the rest of the list over the next few months.

Inflammation and Stress

Going through chronic emotional, mental, and physical stress affects inflammation in the system to a very high degree. When the body is exposed to stress, cortisol levels start to rise.

Cortisol is a steroid hormone that is produced in response to high levels of stress. This may occur from real stressful events, an unhealthy diet, chronic caffeine and stimulant use. Concerning inflammation, the stress reaction that starts to develop to relieve the body from tolerating such circumstances isn't switched off. Chronic stress is tied to chronic inflammation responses. In fact, chronic stress has a negative impact on various body functions. For example, it raises blood pressure and creates hypertension eventually. Chronic high blood pressure also puts blood vessels under a tremendous amount of stress. Strokes and heart failures are common phenomenon in people suffering from chronic inflammation because of inflammatory responses triggered non-stop.

Stress can really "eat" you! The hormone cortisol (stress hormone) actually eats away at your own body tissue to produce energy. It destroys ligament and cartilage tissue. Thus, it is vital to learn ways to deal with high stress levels so that you avoid chronic inflammation. Some valuable relaxation methods include:

- Yoga/Meditation
- Consuming healthy and nutrient-dense foods
- Learning ways to keep emotional tranquility
- Breathing exercises
- Mild exercise

Movement Decreases Inflammation

You must exercise. It is not an option to skip this critical aspect. You may try to justify not exercising because you already work hard at work, you already chase the kids around the house, or you already work in the garden. All of these activities are a good start to movement, but for many individuals, more variety is necessary. I have a very physical job but if I do not weight train and practice yoga my joints suffer. I accumulate pain and increase the chance of injury. That being said, you can turn normal chores and activities into exercise. The overall idea is to be as active as possible in multiple disciplines in order to stay healthy.

I would like everyone to remember one quote: MOVEMENT IS LIFE!

Your assignment this month is to move every day. You may choose anything from the following list:

Vacuum your House

Sweep/Mop your house

Walk the dog for a half hour

Go to the gym

Go for a 15-minute walk/ jog

Yard work

Sports

Important note, over-exercising will increase pain. However, I am not thinking that is a problem for the vast majority of you. That's just for the people that weight train or run 6-7 days a week. The overtraining individual may need to dial it back to allow for recovery between exercises to decrease inflammation. This may involve more rest days or more days working at a lower intensity/ heart rate. If you have the ability to track your heart rate, you should stick to this equation. Find 220 minus your age. Multiply that by .55 and .80. This will give you your range for "fat burning" exercise. Many fatigued or burnt out athletes may even have to reduce to .70 or 70% of the 220 minus age equation until their system can catch up. My personal range lately is 105 to 135, a low range because I have been burning the candle at both ends and my exercise capacity is low as a result. If I go above this range, I get an exercise induced headache because it's too intense. That is how I found my limit. Many high intensity programs put the heart rate above 80% (or the 0.8 in the equation). This is past fat burning and is where exercise can get inflammatory if done without proper rest periods. We will discuss how to exercise in this range later (it is call High Intensity Interval Training).

With the exception of overtraining situations, movement inhibits pain and decreases inflammation. Movement of the spine releases a molecule called GABA; GABA regulates pain perception. Exercise releases endorphins; more endorphins help us tolerate pain. Exercise increases oxygen, which every cell needs. It also helps you trust your muscles and joints so they do not waste away for fear of pain. Exercise can create changes in the spinal cord and motor cortex that help control pain in the brain. The mechanisms are endless.

We will go into more specifics on exercise later but the main point really is the Fitbit mentality: get your steps in. That is the most important component to exercise. That is how you lose weight. That is how you feel better. I have experimented with this, in a full morning of house cleaning I burned more calories and got more steps than I did at the gym. While I love exercise, just simply moving really is the most important. So don't feel guilty if you miss the gym or your workout was sub-par, be satisfied in knowing that at least you created movement, or pick one of the other activities above to add. In the popular seminar called "living to 100" simple movement everyday was one of the top 5 components to a long and healthy life. They specifically say that it doesn't have to be intense exercise. You just have to do productive physical activity daily.

Being Social

Speaking of living, part of the human experience is being social. Your other assignment this month is attending 2 social engagements per week that are unrelated to work. Now, this may seem extremely simple to some, but I assure that for others this may be a struggle. Enjoying time with friends is extremely important to your mental health. This can also influence other factors such as digestion. I suggest another great book called The Slow Down Diet to learn more about the food-psychology connection. The main point is this, when we are relaxed and enjoying time with friends we decrease stress and increase our rest and digest system. This can lead to increased food absorption. Did you know that in France, workers take approximately 2 hours to enjoy lunch with friends, during the work week! In many other countries, it is even typical to share a wine or beer. We are just too wound up on our all work, high stress environment in this country.

The increase in technology has also walled us off more from our friends/family. Many would rather stay home and watch Netflix than be social. While we all need a little R&R and at times, always avoiding social situations will negatively affect your brain. You will not feel as satisfied, depression will increase, and the most obvious-you will likely feel lonely! So get off your cell, computer and TV and go meet your crew at a local hang out.

Loneliness has huge implications in pain perception as well as inflammation. I know I always had the most health issues when I lived far away from home. In times that you feel secluded, you feel more pain from inflammation. This is one of many reasons night shift workers have more pain, they see less of their social circle. Socially isolated people tend to suffer and even die earlier. Loneliness depresses the immune system, not just your mood. It decreases immune cells like your natural killer cells that fight viruses. This makes you more prone to illnesses like cold and flu. I know my husband also got the flu more when he lived out west away from family.

If the chemical explanation of being social does not convince you, think about humans basic needs. We will reference the psychologist Maslow's hierarchy. The main needs are food, water, rest, safety and shelter. The next level of human needs is intimate relationships, friends, family, and sense of connection. It is love and belonging. It is necessary for life. They are fundamental needs for our psyche.

Pills for Inflammation Control

Anti-inflammatory substances for pain relief feature NSAIDS such as Ibuprofen and Aspirin. Other substances are the ones called corticosteroids (cortisone, prednisone), and numbing pain relievers. Typically, anti-inflammatory drug substances demonstrate exaggerated side effects. For instance, the consumption of cortisone for extended periods of time can lead to serious problems with bone strength and integrity. These patients will get bone breaks so easily it will not require trauma. Those experiencing asthma symptoms should also seek an alternative treatment option due to negative side effects from anti-inflammatory drugs. Many chronic takers of NSAIDS also develop stomach ulcers and internal bleeding because of the mucus development blocking attributes of these pharmaceuticals. The gastric wall is further exposed to stomach acid in those who consume NSAIDS for longer periods of time to fight inflammation.

As stated before, your pain is not a deficiency in pain killers. It may be another nutritional deficiency or just from creating too much inflammation in your body.

The most common-sense way to control chronic inflammation is to avoid the triggers we have discussed. We can also change our treatment approach. Instead of prescribing synthetic drugs to hinder inflammatory reactions, I suggest the use of vitamins/nutrients and lifestyle changes. While it's true that some vitamins and nutrients have powerful antioxidant and anti-inflammatory properties, they do not shut off beneficial healing cells like some prescriptions may (such as steroids).

For more complex individuals, further evaluation needs to be performed to find out the exact leading cause of inflammation. It's not holistic or beneficial to only treat the symptoms. It is important to pinpoint the leading culprit of inflammation. For many individuals, more than the top 5 factor will need to be considered. Many patients will need blood testing to identify cause. There are certain markers for inflammation.

Blood Tests for Inflammation

One of the common blood tests to find out inflammation is CRP (C-reactive protein test). This test can pinpoint any heightened levels of the protein, which is considered a sign of inflammation. In several situations when an individual suffers from chronic inflammation which leads to a serious disorder like cancer, arthritis, diabetes, heart failure, or connective tissue (muscle, joints, bones, ligaments) disease, CRP levels are elevated.

Homocysteine amounts in the blood can also be determined from blood testing. Homocysteine is an acid that is produced by the system physiologically when we consume excessive amounts of red meat. When homocysteine levels are abnormally elevated, the person is a high risk of developing heart problems, atherosclerosis, heart failure, stroke and even Alzheimer's disease.

There are many factors that can increase these inflammatory markers. It can be from diet, allergies, leaky gut, deficiencies, lack of exercise, or many of the factors discussed in this book.

The Gut Connection

Researchers and medical experts keep on examining the leading cause of inflammation. With so many contributing factors and issues linked to our diets, it's no surprise that gut inflammation has a vital role to play here. That is why we mentioned food sensitivities in the previous chapter. We will be discussing many more gut factors as we progress. For example, leaky gut plays a huge role in inflammation. It is likely the top player. Leaky gut allows toxins into the blood, stimulates the immune response, allows chronic gut infections, and decreases absorption. Leaky gut can encompass all 5 inflammation causes: food, toxins, bugs, trauma, and hormones. That being said, leaky gut management is a complicated process. We will start by discussing the two main causes of gut integrity loss: Gluten and Dairy.

Assignments

Attend 2 social engagements per week (non-work related)

Start the baseline anti-inflammatory diet, eliminate top 5 offenders

Move every day

Month 3

Team Sports, Gluten, and Accountability

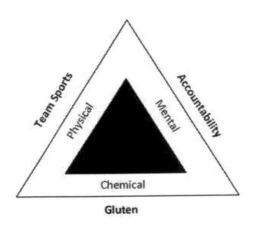

My Experience

I stopped athletics when I went to college. I was never so lost in my life. I threatened to quit or change schools' multiple times because I was not happy or satisfied. Fast forward to graduate school. I found Crossfit. This was like gym class and team sports combined for adults. It changed my life and it increased my potential at school. I was a happier human and was more productive in other areas when I had athletics and sports back in my life. I only wish I had tried to find it sooner. Competitive sports make you more able to handle competition in all areas of your life. That edge also pushes you to get a better workout. I have always performed better in life when very active at a sport.

Team sports, and athletics in general, are a huge area for creating happiness in your life. It also provides unparalleled levels of accountability. One of the main reasons I show up to Crossfit is because the owner is my neighbor, my husband goes, and my sister goes. All these people, as well as the other members I have befriended, are dependable for harassing me if I miss a week. Accountability is needed for workout consistency. Team atmospheres are the best way to acquire it.

Team Sports

One of the questions on the patient intake form in my office is, "how often do you exercise? " Patients almost always view this question as synonymous with how many days they visit the gym or the treadmill. Most forget to include team sports, hiking, outdoor activities, and games. As mentioned in the previous chapter, getting off your butt doesn't always have to mean really intense exercise. Healthy people will engage in many disciplines of physical activity in their life. Movement is life. Move as much as you can each day, regardless of activity.

It's funny to me how healthy kids are without having a membership at a gym? Why is that? It comes down to one word, PLAY. As adults, we forget to play, to learn new things, to have fun moving our bodies. We look at the gym as an hour of pure misery that needs to be accomplished to stay healthy. We pay hundreds of dollars for our kids to join gymnastics, hockey, and soccer but don't want to spend more than $10 a month on our own fitness. This paradigm needs to change. If you pay $300 a month on kid's tennis lessons, you deserve to spend some money on some athletic fun for yourself as well.

Options for Play

Team sports are one way adults can play. They can let out their competitive spirit, interact with others, joke around, and even break a sweat in the process. I don't even care if its beer league softball or bowling, team sports are an important area of health. This is especially true for athletes; people that played college sports or were really competitive in high school. For these individuals, sports were a defining portion of their identity as it was for me. It is dangerous to lose that as an adult.

For those on the not so athletic side, I believe you can still find the sport that is right for you. Learning new things is an integral part of health. Many sports are divided into ability levels, such as tennis. That way you can stay active, have fun, and not worry about being a bit clumsy. Even some martial arts gyms, running clubs, dance groups, boot camps, or weight training clubs have a fun group atmosphere for those new to athletics.

Non-Sport Play

Arrange social activities. Find group fun that involves something besides sitting at a bar. Golf, dance, throw a ball around, etc. Find something local like axe throwing, paintball, kayaking, skiing, or shooting.

Schedule time outdoors. Being outside stimulates the brain, grounds you energetically, increases oxygen, and more. Get off the beaten path and adventure. We will discuss this in depth in later chapters.

Play with pets/children. They know better how to have fun than any of us do. I mean, do you see how ecstatic your dog is when you get home?

Quit being an old lazy bum and chase your niece the next time she asks to play tag!

Benefits of Play

Relieve stress. Play is fun and can trigger the release of endorphins, the body's natural feel-good chemicals. Endorphins promote an overall sense of well-being and can even temporarily relieve pain.

Improve brain function. Play cognitive games. Get into twister, yard games (corn hole, yard golf, yard darts, croquet), board games, charades, card games, escape rooms, arts and crafts, sports, etc. The social interaction of playing with family and friends can also help ward off depression.

Stimulate the mind and boost creativity. Young children often learn best when they are playing—and that principle applies to adults, as well. You'll learn a new task better when it's fun and you're in a relaxed and playful mood. Play can also stimulate your imagination, helping you adapt and problem solve.

Retain your youth. My grandparents spend time in a retirement community that has everything from tennis, long distance biking, Spanish classes, computer classes, sewing clubs, to parties. There is no doubt in my mind that this keeps them younger. I used to always brag to friends about the fun activities I would do with them from hiking to museums to crafts. They never sit still and are always learning new things. My Grandma picked up tennis at the age of 70 seriously. Keep learning and keep playing, it keeps you young.

Team sports, play, clubs/groups, and fun family time also move us into our other topic this month which is accountability.

Accountability is the glue that ties commitment to the result.

Accountability looks different to everyone. Accountability means that you are honest with yourself and responsible for what you do. You are responsible for you own health. As with most things in this book, you have to find what works for you. For certain individuals, it is better to have someone else hold them accountable. This is when we require coaches. A few ideas are: personal trainers, health coaches, fitness groups, small class size group training, sticking with a buddy, making changes as a family/couple, tracking with a calendar or journal, etc.

There are also some goal oriented ways to stay accountable such as buying a vacation if you reach your goal, allowing yourself a new wardrobe when you hit your goal weight, placing bets with friends/family colleagues. I remember my uncle doing a weight loss bet with his friend some time ago. The bet was for $1,000 each. They told me the stakes had to be high enough for them to put the effort in because $50 just wouldn't do it.

Putting some skin in the game.

That brings me to one more accountability technique: investing. For better or for worse, many of us are driven by money. With myself and many patients I find we try harder after we have put a great deal of money into our health. For example, I am more likely to quit a diet that I just read a book about than a cleanse I spend $300 on. If I bought $300 worth of supplements you bet I am going to complete that program. Some of you may need to buy that 6 month membership up front or go for the expensive meal plans to actually reach your goals because you don't want to waste the money of not using what you already paid for.

You become like those you surround yourself with most.

I am a firm believer in this principle. I have lived with many different people and have noticed many changes in my health based on these situations. One relationship in graduate school was a great example of the negativity that can overcome you. I dated a dude that would criticize me for eating healthy. He always asked for sweets and was convinced that glucose was the only viable energy source. He thought my digestive disturbances were a myth and did not believe in food allergies or intolerances. He accused me of cheating on him if I spent too much time at the gym, convinced I must be sleeping with my Crossfit trainer. Well, thank goodness I had joined Crossfit and that gave me the strength to escape this downward spiral. I was the fattest I had been in my life and felt like shit all the time.

Fast forward a year, I moved in with an old college friend. We would share cooking. We empowered each other to exercise. We kept on eye on sugar consumption. We would hike and travel and had a blast. At this point, I achieved the thinnest I had been since high school. I was excelling at Crossfit and felt great in my own skin. I bought a super skimpy bikini and life was good.

Now I also live in a positive healthful environment. I found a wonderful man that supports my diet and exercise lifestyle. He even pushes me to advance my health daily. I have a health minded family and sister with similar philosophies to my own. It definitely keeps me accountable and empowers me to stick to my efforts.

It is important to find your people. If you want to be athletic and positive and healthful, find other people that act this way. If you surround yourself with sick and lazy individuals then that is what you will become.

Unfortunately, this at times means taking time away from family or loved ones at first. They may not understand your new lifestyle. Unfortunately, those that are sinking want others to drown with them. However, once you stick to your healthful path long enough, you will become a beacon of inspiration for others. Have you ever heard "hustle until your haters ask if you are hiring?" People will likely discourage you at first, particularly those close to you (unless they are already on a health path themselves). Eventually, the haters will ask what you are doing to make such great progress. Then you will be the one coaching them.

Start with your family. It is easier to make changes if you implement them as a household. If you have a certain food related discomfort or disease, it is likely your kids or family does as well. The apple doesn't fall far from the tree. Now, I do not want to hear excuses such as "my kids won't eat it" or "my husband will complain." If you do the grocery shopping, they eat what you buy, simple as that. Give them an education on why your family will benefit from the changes and if they still give you flack, then say "suck it up buttercup!" My husband was extremely hesitant about starting the keto diet. He thought it would not fit well with his physiology, he has trouble keeping on weight and had part of his guts removed due to an accident bull riding in younger years. That is not a joke. When there were no carbs left in the house though he admitted to feeling improved energy and the best digestion in years. One of the main carbohydrate sources people eat are gluten containing grains, specifically wheat. Going on low to no carbohydrate diets help many people simply due to the diet lacking this substance. There are many reasons gluten can be harmful and they are not all allergies. Gluten causes inflammation by multiple mechanisms. My household feels better without it. Let's check out the reasons why.

The Gluten Problem

The first food to get out of your house is gluten. Everyone in your home may not be sensitive to it, but we will discuss its many negative effects regardless of allergy or not. We talk a lot about inflammatory foods in this book. Food allergies cause inflammation. Most food containing gluten is inflammatory, and filled with sugar. If you want to eat an anti-inflammatory diet you must eliminate known food allergies.

The top 5 are

1. Gluten
2. Dairy
3. Soy
4. Corn
5. Eggs

As discussed in chapter 3 there are many reasons why you react poorly to food. Your body is the best doctor to diagnose what foods are right or wrong for you. However, there are times when we are not quite in tuned with our bodies yet. Some people are so used to feeling terrible, that they do not recognize bad reactions or they blame the problem on the weather, their bed/pillow, stress, driving, sitting, age, etc. Therefore, I would like to spend some time explaining the negative effect of gluten seems it is the top offender. That being said, allergies/reactions can be to anything. I had a patient recently get lab work done that indicated extreme allergies to beef and bananas. These are not foods I would have predicted for an allergy. She eliminated these two foods and drastically decreased her arthritis pain to the point where she quit worrying about needing a knee replacement surgery. Therefore, gluten and dairy are not always the answer but I will give them at least an 80% likelihood on being the cause of inflammation and allergies.

What Is Gluten?

Gluten is not a protein itself but rather a protein composite, which means it is composed of several different proteins. The primary proteins giving gluten its utility in baking and its difficulty in health are glutenin and gliadin (in wheat), secalin (in rye) and hordein (from barley). Gluten is the binding agent that gives food a chewy quality. Ever notice how gluten free products crumble to dust? That is why.

The tricky part of gluten is that it tends to contaminate other grains as well. Oats are often harvested and processed alongside wheat and thus may be cross-contaminated. In some rare cases, even oats guaranteed to be gluten-free may trigger cross-reactivity in celiac patients. So, extremely sensitive patients need to be wary of this factor.

You can see how tracking down gluten containing vs. gluten free food can be tricky? That's why most products simply say gluten friendly instead. It is hard to commit with 100% certainty that a product is not contaminated. You may reference the appendix for a list of gluten containing ingredients.

One key point to consider is that gluten is in more foods and products than you may realize. If you think removing gluten from your diet involves just avoiding bread and baked goods, I'm afraid you're mistaken. It is not surprising that gluten can cause problems in everyone when we add it to everything we eat including non-grain products. Our system is on gluten overdose. It is even in some lunch meat. Why would you ever expect that? It is often used in sauces, flavorings, flavor enhancers and even as a binder or filler in medications, vitamins and supplements. They hide the shit in everything imaginable. Adapting a true gluten-free diet requires more than just removing wheat products from your lifestyle.

What Is Gluten Intolerance?

First you must separate gluten intolerance into three distinct categories: Celiac Disease, Gluten Sensitivity and a Wheat Allergy.

Celiac Disease occurs when the proteins in gluten (glutenin and gliadin, but primarily gliadin) trigger your immune system to overreact with strong and unusual antibodies. Over time, the reaction caused by these antibodies wears down the villi that line the walls of your intestine. The villi, which are finger-like protrusions along the wall of your small intestine, grab and absorb nutrients as foods pass through your lower digestive tract. As this autoimmune response slowly flattens the villi, you become less and less able to process any nutrition from your food. This may lead to serious mal-absorption issues and stunted growth. Celiac disease also triggers inflammation of the intestinal wall. The combination of absorption-killing villous atrophy and inflammation sets off a domino-effect of increasingly serious health problems.

Celiac disease is also one cause for leaky gut syndrome (discussed at length later). Leaky gut may cause rashes, joint pain, seasonal allergies, IBS and more.

Wheat allergy symptoms create the second category. A wheat allergy is a histamine response to wheat, much like a peanut allergy or hay fever. Some people experience hives while others might experience stomach pain. I have heard the stomach pain described as a stomach migraine. This is where you get a typical allergic response.

Gluten Sensitivity (GS) is currently a little more difficult to pinpoint. Basically, individuals who suffer from GS suffer similarly to people with Celiac Disease, but the blood test and biopsy used to identify and diagnose celiac disease is negative. Gluten Sensitive patients also test negative for a wheat allergy. This is important because this leads to these patients problems being neglected due to insufficient tests. GS may be due to reactions to other components of grains such as lectins. Lectins are a coating on many grains, beans and nuts that one may be sensitive too. Others are sensitive to FODMAPS (different plant sugars) which are high in grains. Some are just sensitive to yeast/mold used for some baked goods. I will say that I am reactive to mostly the yeast/mold/FODMAPS part of gluten. On single exposure, I do not notice a reaction. However, if I overdose I will be swelled up and miserable. I also occasionally get the swelled up eyes if my mold exposure is too high. I will never go back to New Orleans for that reason, too much mold. The only way to confidently diagnose GS is through elimination diets. Quit all consumption of the food for 3 weeks then add it back in and observe symptoms for the next 4-5 days. As I state frequently, you are your best doctor.

Recent research and current gluten intolerance statistics suggest that 10% to 15% of the population may suffer from some form of intolerance to this troublesome protein complex, and yet the vast majority of these individuals have not yet been properly diagnosed. Furthermore, we now know even patients who test negative for celiac disease may suffer from some form of undiagnosed non-celiac gluten intolerance. One Italian study found that 3/100 children tested positive for celiac disease.

What Are Gluten Intolerance Symptoms?

Here is a list of possible gluten intolerance symptoms. Now some may seem far-fetched. Remember, you are what you eat. If your body hates what you eat, it hates itself and will attack with inflammation.

Abdominal Pain and Cramping
Alternating Bouts of Diarrhea and Constipation
Anemia
Arthritis
Attention Deficit Disorder (ADD)
Back pain
Bloating
Bone Density Loss
Brittle Nails
Canker sores
Constipation
Stunted Growth
Depression
Anxiety
Dry Hair
Diabetes
Diarrhea
Edema
Fatigue
Malodorous Stools
Grayish Stools
Hair Loss (Alopecia)
Headaches and Migraines
Hypoglycemia
Infertility
Joint pain
Juvenile Idiopathic Arthritis
Lactose intolerance
Nausea
Numbness or tingling
Osteoporosis
Peripheral Neuropathy
Sjogren's Disease
Steatorrhea
Teeth and Gum Problems
Vitamin and Mineral deficiencies
Vomiting
Unexplained Weight loss
Urticaria

I hope this gluten intolerance checklist helps you, but again, do not try to diagnose yourself from a list. These symptoms could stem from many other root causes. Talk to your functional medicine doctor to help you differentiate.

What Is Celiac Disease?

Celiac disease is when you have a lot of gluten antibodies to point where your body reacts to the villi in your gut, an autoimmune condition. It is diagnosed if there are positive antibodies to a part of gluten, to human tissue transglutaminase, and the intestinal wall. If the immune system is so badly altered by this protein that it makes your body attack itself, it must be avoided at all costs. Usually antibodies are present to protect the body and fight infections. Whenever the immune system goes out of check like this is makes us more prone to more serious conditions such as cancer. Many undiagnosed celiac patients end up with cancer, Alzheimer's, ataxia, or other severe conditions. 7/8 patients are misdiagnosed. Not only that, other allergies (besides t gluten) can destroy intestinal villi. In fact, even just the glycophosphates (round-up) that wheat is treated with can do it. Another component of gluten that cause allergies is gluteomorphin (a morphine like addiction) that makes coming off gluten like a drug withdrawal.

Symptoms can be anything from digestive distress, brain fog, swelling and pain in joints, hypothyroid, inability to grow, infertility, to heart disease. Food allergies do not always have gut related symptoms!! In fact many do not! 1/133 people have celiac but only 35% have typical GI symptoms and you can develop them at any point throughout life. As it has often gone misdiagnosed or undiagnosed in the past, you may have gluten intolerance in your family and not realize it. If there is gluten intolerance or celiac in your family, get rid of it now. You are likely to develop some level of issue with it later in life.

Thankfully, people are becoming more sensitive and aware of gluten intolerance in children so gluten intolerance symptoms in children are now much more likely to be diagnosed than they were just ten years ago. Gluten intolerance symptoms in adults, however, are still generally blamed on other conditions such as ulcerative colitis, Crohn's disease, lactose intolerance, irritable bowel syndrome and yeast intolerance. Hint: gluten is a root cause for many people with these conditions. And because adults too often grow accustomed to some discomforts as they age, celiac disease symptoms in adults often go undiagnosed and untreated.

As discussed, you are your best doctor. Not all tests are dependable. Allergy testing is dependent on the immune system at that moment. For example, I had my allergies tested in undergrad. We all know undergrad is not the healthiest point in life. I tested allergic to the earth. It looked like I needed to move into a bubble. Fast forward to postgraduate school, the only allergy that came back positive was gelatin. Different times in life, different allergies, different immune system.

Adults experiencing unexplained joint pain, anemia, infertility or osteoporosis should discuss the possibility of gluten intolerance with their primary care physician. Your gut changes every 4 days. With that amount of variance, food sensitivities also tend to change or evolve. For example, if you get leaky gut temporarily from a food poisoning incident that may be enough to send your immune system into a new food allergy developing. You do not have to have an allergy permanently. Allergies are dependent on the state of your immune system and therefore can come and go throughout life.

Common Testing vs Complete Testing

Remember how I said labs are useless? Well some people still need a piece of paper to tell them what is right for their body so I will discuss a variety of testing.

You can react to many components of gluten/wheat. Most tests only look at one or two antibodies and completely ignore digestion deficiencies. You can test IgG, IgA, and IgE antibodies. You can test for at least 10 different components of the gluten protein. You can also test for auto-immune antibodies. The typical lab only tests IgG. So you can see that many testing components are often missed.

Another point of discrepancy on tests is if you have already gone gluten free. My sister had gluten problems before it got popular. We had no idea what was wrong with her. Eventually we learned about Celiac and thought that it fit. However, she had adopted a gluten-free diet long before that. Since she has been GF for so long, her intestinal villi was intact, giving her a negative diagnosis. Though the doctors did tell her she may still have the disease, she just had been GF for so long her villi may have already recovered. If you do not consume a food it will likely not show up on tests. Similar discrepancies can happen on antibody tests. I would find a doctor that will order from Cyrex labs if you are concerned about test results.

Gluten may not be the only problem

The round-up used to treat many grains may be the root cause of many food intolerances. The substance in round-up called glycophosphate causes digestive disturbances in healthy individuals. This even affects animals. I worked in a barn where the horses were developing food intolerances and auto-immune diseases as a result of glyphosate laden hay.

Also, mold in storage in silos causes an immune reaction in patients. Many people are reactive to molds.

The way we process grains also plays a role. Deamidation exposes us to more components of gluten. This process is used to make gluten more soluble for cooking. These exposed components are often what we react to. This is why some gluten sensitive individuals can tolerate sprouted grains such as ezekiels. These sprouted grains are not processed the same as conventional grains.

You can see then why gluten problems have become more prevalent. We have changed how we use and how we process this product.

Why am I gluten free and feel no better?

Many will "go gluten-free" and not notice a difference. However, these 5 sneaky mechanisms may be holding you back from feeling that allergen-free bliss.

1. Leaky gut - Reactivity against many foods can cause or be a result of leaky gut. This is a condition that causes leakage of food into the bloodstream causing an immune reaction.

2. Missing hidden sources - listed in appendix. Remember, even a thumb sized portion of gluten can affect your immune system. Elimination has to be complete.

3. FODMAPS- FODMAPS stands for sugar to oversimplify. You may be fructose (sugar) intolerant. If you are reactive to sugars such as this, you may need to be grain free entirely, not just gluten free. You will also need to monitor other sugar sources closely such as fruit. I will mention that this is where I find myself. I did feel much better going GF, but it was not enough. I did not reach my full gut potential until ditching all grains. If I expose myself to gluten, I do not have any crazy allergic reactions. I will get gradually inflamed, get joint pain, my face gets puffy, etc. When I am grain free, these all disappear.

4. Gluten can stay in the gut for up to 6 months -Some may need help with digestive enzymes to eliminate the stagnant proteins in gut.

5. Gluten cross reactors (listed in appendix): the immune system looks at these foods and sees them as gluten, so it attacks because they look so similar. Cross reactivity can apply to our own organ tissue as well. For example, thyroid tissue and gluten tissue look similar to your immune system. So gluten can end up destroying your thyroid if your antibodies are tagging both for disposal. I like to think of certain immune cells as blind pac men, like the game. They eat any color of ghosts because they all seem the same. However, one color of ghost may have been gluten and the other thyroid.

Assignments

Adopt Gluten Free Lifestyle

Join a Team or Club

Find an Accountability buddy (family member, friend, trainer, journal, class etc.)

Month 4

Sugar, High Intensity Interval Training, and Community

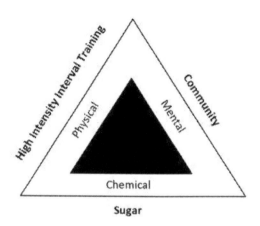

My Experience

When I started seeing Dr. Huff, my functional medicine doctor, I had wellness blood work done for the first time. One of the first things he told me was that I had pre-diabetes. I was mortified. I was a normal weight. I was exercising 6-7 days a week. I watched what I ate and included all my fruits and veggies. How could I have diabetes?

Turns out, just because I was eating "healthy" did not mean I was eating healthy amounts of sugar. I learned that I was eating way too much fruit. I drank sugary alcoholic drinks on weekends. I had high carb/sugar snacks to keep up with my workouts. I found out that my sugar intake was way too high. I just had never considered that as being a problem seems I tried to avoid desserts and lattes.

As it turns out, I could not out-exercise a bad diet. I was doing HIIT exercise as we will discuss. HIIT is the best exercise to help blood sugar, but reducing sugar intake is still needed to fix physiology. I had to cut my sugar way lower than anticipated to fix my blood work numbers.

The Sugar Problem

Blood sugar dysregulation is one mechanism that contributes to all metabolic disease present today. It is of utmost importance when healing anything from hormones, heart disease, cancer, diabetes to gut discomforts. Sadly, the average American consumes 2-3 pounds of sugar on a weekly basis. The number may seem exaggerated at first, but that is because the majority of sugar consumed is not in cakes or cookies but rather hidden as additives. Sugar is highest in our beverages and hidden in everything from ketchup to skim milk. Sugar intake has risen from 5lbs. a year in the 19th century to 135 lbs. per year in this one. It is important to consider that up until the early 20th century, cancer and heart problem rates were totally absent. This blatant association has been backed-up by late scientific evidence that demonstrates that the more sugar someone takes, the higher the risk of developing health problems later in their lives. From elevated cholesterol levels to lower immune activity, sugar has a detrimental impact on our system. Yes, excess sugar increases cholesterol! Not what you thought right? Sugar directly increases LDL (bad cholesterol) production.

Sugar and Immunity

A study performed during the 1970s, found that white blood cells required Vitamin C to expel out bacteria, viruses, and other intruders. White blood cells need 50X the amount of Vitamin C as normal cells. Due to the fact that both Vitamin C and sugar have similar chemical forms; they antagonize each other when blood sugar levels get raised in the bloodstream. They rival each other to penetrate the cell. Therefore, when there are higher amounts of sugar present in the bloodstream, due to eating high GI foods, this will allow fewer amounts of Vitamin C to penetrate the cell. When we take high amounts of sugar, the immune system function will come to a sticky end.

We are all familiar with how vitamin C impacts the common cold. This principle also applies to inflammatory disorders like diabetes, cancer, heart problems, and asthma. Many countries use intravenous vitamin C as a cancer therapy in fact. The common denominator here is the high intake of sugar destroying our immune system and making us sick. We need to decrease sugar consumption so that vitamin C has a chance to do its job.

Cancer Feeds on Sugar

In the early 1930s, German Scientist Otto Warburg, has been awarded a Nobel Prize for being the first to discover the fluctuating energy metabolism of cancer cells as opposed to that of healthy cells. The final finding emerging from his trials was that cancer cells use sugar at a much more elevated pace than normal healthy cells. The more sugar exists in the system, the more it is taken by the cells of the body. So in other words, the sugar actually is a source of food for cancer cells and can

75

contribute to their spread and development at a later stage. Cancer cells have at least 4 times the number of sugar receptors as normal cells.

As emerging from the above study, cancer treatment protocols nowadays are aiming to control blood sugar levels by aiming at low sugar/carbohydrate diets.

Sugar and Mental Health

Sugar has a detrimental effect on the central nervous system and mental health. First off, balanced blood glucose is required for transport of neurotransmitter precursors across the blood brain barrier. For example: tryptophan is used to make serotonin (feel good hormone). Tryptophan cannot get to the brain to make serotonin without these healthy glucose channels. You can see how low blood sugar could actually cause depression eh? Sugar also inhibits growth hormones that ultimately trigger long-term inflammation. The inflammation process hinders the activity of the immune system and leads to mental/brain issues. Long-term inflammation in the system is triggered by high intake of sugar, which suppresses the normal activity of the immune system and makes it lose its power to fight back. Additionally, sugar leads to a fast spike in adrenaline levels which triggers episodes of induced stress, anxiety, hyperactivity, and struggle to maintain focus (ADD/ADHD).

Sugar on the Brain

When there is a high sugar intake, some changes emerge in the brain. Animal trials demonstrated alterations in the dopamine levels of the brain, emerge after the intake of sugar. Sugar has similar dopamine effects on the brain as cocaine. This neurologic response makes sugar elimination very difficult. Some will have extreme withdrawal symptoms from reducing sugar similar to a drug detox.

The sugar addiction will also make you dislike other healthy foods. For example, those with sugar dependence hate vegetables. Many also have a dislike for protein. That is because vegetables and protein have little to no sugar. If the dependence on the sugar flavor is broken, these foods will become appetizing. This happens often with kids. Kid products are full of sugar and most of kids' protein is breaded. This makes them hate protein and many health disparities come with that such as growing pains. This sounds untrue but your brain creates a response to foods it is used too. If your brain deems a food safe due to repeat exposure that did not kill it, it says that that food tastes good. If you give you brain a repeat exposure to healthy foods, it will like them more. I can honestly say the first time I gave up sugar I thought I would die. After a month of powering through the detox, I tried a Reese's cup. I spit it out. I no longer appreciate any milk chocolate. It is too sweet. I can only handle dark, my taste buds changed by changing my exposure and physiology.

Sugar and Fatigue (Adrenal Health)

A common syndrome that occurs with blood sugar instability is Adrenal Fatigue. The Adrenals are a gland located on the kidneys involved in you "fight or flight" response. However, it does much more. Adrenals are in charge of "sweet, salty, sex." That may sound quirky, but it is quite true. Adrenals produce male and female hormones such as estrogen and testosterone. They also produce hormones that balance salt and minerals. Lastly, they help control blood sugar and stress with cortisol. Cortisol or Adrenaline is released in stressful situations such as running from a tiger (fight or flight). They both increase blood sugar. This is great if you are actually running from a tiger; however, most of us are not. We are only living stressful lives and constantly releasing this hormone that increases blood sugar until it gets burnt out (adrenal fatigue). When this happens, it is difficult to maintain blood sugar. But Cortisol is not the only hormone affected. The "salty sex" hormones are diminished as well, and this may be taken literally. A fatigued adrenal will diminish sex drive as well as male/female hormones. It will also mess with salt balance producing either dehydration chronically or swelling. So, I am sure you can imagine the symptoms adrenal fatigue produces between "Hanger" or hungry/angry, low libido, weight loss resistance, insomnia, hormone balance, chronic fatigue, high blood pressure and dehydration to list a few. To aid with these symptoms there are protocols delineated the appendix. All in all, decreasing sugar is the key to controlling all of the aforementioned conditions.

Where is the sugar?

It is very difficult to stay under the American Heart Association's recommendation of 25g of sugar a day without taking added/hidden sugars into account. Sugar is sneakily hidden in so many kinds of foods that we have no other option than to read the list of ingredients in every food label to find it. There are three general rules when it comes to deciphering food labels:

No 1: Find out any words ending in -ose e.g. sucralose, fructose, dextrose, etc.

No 2: Look at the Nutrition Facts Label to see how many grams of sugar are in the product

No 3: Anything containing the word syrup. Especially offensive is high fructose corn syrup.

The Glycemic Index

Every carbohydrate is measured by its effect on blood sugar. Often, the amount of sugar in a product is correlated to its GI (glycemic index). This is a 0-100 scale of a foods effect on your body. You may also reference the GI chart in the appendix for a list of such foods. This will help you further discover what foods contain more sugar. For example, many fruits are higher than candy in sugar content. Glycemic index will show you that.

Low glycemic index foods release energy slowly into the system. An increased GI score means that the food drastically spikes sugar and later insulin. When high GI foods are consumed chronically, you will lose insulin sensitivity which makes your blood sugar less stable. You become more prone to fatigue. High GI foods make you crave more caffeine and more sugar in order to try and maintain blood sugar. If you are unable to have a high sugar/caffeine snack, it will be nap time. Low GI foods help keep energy levels stabilized and prevent those infamous sudden sugar spikes which lead to energy crashes throughout the day. Biasing your sugar/carbohydrates to low GI drastically improves health even without full sugar elimination. It also will help decrease inflammation.

How to Balance Blood Sugar

The most obvious way to balance blood sugar is easy, QUIT EATING SUGAR! Since this suggestion is a lot harder than it sounds we will discuss a few more options. As similar to other topics in this book, everyone reacts differently to different foods. This includes sugar and carbohydrates. Sugar is just one type of carbohydrate and they should be viewed as having similar effect on our chemistry. Some people genetically have a lower tolerance. If you have a low tolerance for sugars, you will easily get carb crashes. The best way to measure this is to monitor how you feel after you eat. If you feel you need a nap, you likely overdid it on sugar/carbohydrates, or you just overate in general.

There are many levels of blood sugar dysregulation. The two main trends are hypoglycemic or insulin resistant. Insulin resistant means that your cells are full, full of food and full of energy. Hypoglycemic is the opposite, the cells are starving for energy and are feeling empty. These can be differentiated with on question: Does food/meals give you energy or make you tired? One of your assignments this month is to choose a protocol based on this question. If your blood sugar is balanced you will likely not experience either. If food gives you energy, you are likely on the hypoglycemic range. If food makes you tired, you are likely on the insulin resistance range. If both occur, you are probably on the insulin resistance range and likely headed down the road to diabetes.

If you are truly hypoglycemic, it is likely that you have burnt out adrenals and may follow that protocol listed in the appendix. If you are either mixed or in the insulin resistance phase, fast forward to moderate fasting in appendix or ketogenic diet in chapter 12. I can attest to being in the mixed phase and had a very hard time treating my blood sugar due to misunderstanding. I always figured I was adrenal fatigued, I have every symptom and every practitioner told me so. It wasn't until I was told to treat my adrenal problem as if it were insulin resistance that I made any progress. I went Keto. When I started eating as if I had insulin resistance, my "hunger" feeling drastically reduced. I was able to go longer without eating and I slept through the night more often. So be sure to distinguish which category you belong to or you may not make much progress.

Exercise and Blood Sugar

Exercise is a key component of balancing blood sugar. It will increase insulin sensitivity, which makes our cells better at letting energy in. It will decrease insulin levels, meaning less inflammation and less insulin resistance. It will also decreases blood sugar levels by utilizing the energy for muscles. It increases metabolism. One great form of exercise for this is HIIT (high intensity interval training).

How to Exercise?

It is important to point out the wrong options first. Of course, I believe any movement counts toward getting fit. Movement is life. However, some exercise can cause harm especially if done repetitively the wrong way. Let's examine what most people do at a gym.

The typical female will usually go do 30 minutes to an hour on a treadmill or similar piece of cardio equipment. Some cardio is great, but if that is the only exercise you do 5 days a week, it will make you prone to injury. When you train the same muscle group over and over without variance, you end up with muscular imbalance. Chronic cardio can also destroy hormones and blood sugar. It is very taxing on the adrenals if done at high intensity for long periods (I am not talking about walking here folks.) Now perhaps this same female gets really motivated and tries to add a "barbell blast" kind of class to her schedule for some variance. Awesome! Accept most of these typical female centered classes do not exceed 20 lbs. worth of weight. If muscles are never put under a significant load, there is no reason for them to build. Putting a load on the back actually forces muscle and bone growth. This is very important for osteoporosis prevention.

Now we can take this the opposite direction. I am addicted to lifting weights. I would prefer it be my only form of exercise. However, if I only lift heavy, my knees start to hurt and my shoulders get stiff. I have to add in some cardio and yoga to keep my body healthy and happy. I hope this helps you see that all exercise requires variety. You can even see this in high school athletes that overtrain. Many teenagers are getting ACL surgeries and rotator cuff surgeries from simply overtraining. They get involved in one sport like baseball and play it 8 months of the year for 15 years. Then they end up with shoulder surgery because their trainers/coaches did not make them vary their routine. In fact, lifting weights at a young age with a proficient trainer is the best way to avoid overtraining injury. A gifted trainer will know to have the athlete stabilize other aspects of the joint not already worked during their sport.

The other destructive thing most people do at the gym is to waste time! They spend more time on their cell phone texting between sets or trying to find the best jam to get their workout done. Many people assume you have to spend an hour at the gym. That is just not true. If you eliminate cell phone time you could cut your gym trip in half! The best ways to eliminate wasted time are by doing organized group training, HIIT training, or both. So let's discuss what HIIT means.

What is HIIT (High-Intensity Interval Training)?

High-intensity interval training (HIIT), is a form of interval training, a cardiovascular exercise strategy alternating short periods of intense anaerobic exercise with less intense recovery periods. Though there is no universal HIIT session duration, these intense workouts typically last under 30 minutes, with times varying based on a participant's current fitness level. Some key vernacular for HIIT training are words like EMOM (every minute on the minute), Tabata (20 sec work 10 sec rest), and AMRAMP (as many reps as possible). These are all great words to type into Pinterest when looking for at home workouts. Or, these are formats you will find at a Crossfit gym.

HIIT workouts train and condition both your aerobic and anaerobic energy systems. HIIT workouts get your heart rate up and improve your cardiovascular fitness level while burning more fat and calories in less time. As stated before, 60 minutes on a treadmill is not needed. HIIT can be effective in less than 10 minutes. Don't believe me? Try doing burpees for 7 minutes. I will bet you are sore the next day and out of breath after.

How Is HIIT Done?

Here are instructions to design your own HIIT exercise.

Step 1 - Determine how long you have (5 to 30 minutes). Keep in mind it is good to keep this changing. So if you do 10 min workouts on Monday and Tuesday, try and throw in a 30 minute one later in the week.

Step 2 - Choose your interval scheme. Remember I mentioned EMOM, AMRAMP, Tabata? These can be used or you can simply set a timer and work for 40 secs followed by a 20 second rest, as an example.

Step 3 -Choose your movements. Movements should be variable (starting to see a pattern yet?) I recommend doing some strength, some gymnastic, some speed some flexibility, and some coordination movements. I will give an example. On Monday I did burpees for speed, squats for strength, bird dogs for flexibility, pull ups for gymnastics and box jumps for coordination. Once you choose your movements, be sure to warm up the areas to be exercised for 3-4 minutes.

Step 4 -Execute. Examples of different movements are:

Cardio - running, jump rope, jumping jacks, biking, swimming

Strength - powerlifting movements (squats, deadlifts, bench press) olympic weight lifting (power cleans, snatch, jerk)

Gymnastics -pull up, handstand, ring rows, muscle up, jungle gyms, rock climbing

Coordination-wall ball, speed rope ladder, fast feet, ball toss, toe touches, burpees

Balance -single leg or single arm exercises, balance ball exercises, holding balance postures

Flexibility - Yoga will be discussed in later chapters but stretching is great post exercise

What Are The Benefits Of HIIT?

Applying HIIT is truly the most effective way to workout. Some of the benefits of HIIT training are: promotes HGH production (human growth hormone), boost metabolism, improves strength and stamina, improves overall health, promotes fat loss, less gym time, and improved blood sugar. One of the greatest advantages of using HIIT is known as the afterburn effect. Which is also known as EPOC (excess post-exercise oxygen consumption). This is when you increase your metabolism and burn more calories for up to 24 hours after training.

Who can do HIIT?

HIIT is great for everyone because you are always putting in YOUR best effort and YOUR highest intensity. Your capacity will improve the longer you train. You could do the same workout over and over and still get a great workout because once you get more proficient, you go faster, which still produces a great effect. Of course, this is all based on the effort you put in. Example: That 7 minutes of burpees I mentioned. The first time you try it you may get 25 repetitions in. You may be exhausted at this point. Now fast forward a year, You would probably be doing 50 or 60 reps. See? Same workout but everyone can do it to their own personal capacity.

The great thing about most gyms that incorporate HIIT is that you are doing small group training. This allows you to compete, meet new people, and stay accountable. It helps you develop a sense of community while incorporating a workout routine. Going to a similar class time each day can really create a friend group of like minded people.

Community

A sense of community is the #1 factor involved when studying how people live to 100 years old. There are many ways to create a community that is meaningful to you. People tend to find their community in family, church, clubs, teams, volunteer groups, etc. Community is by definition a unified body of individuals with common interests or goals. You must find this group for yourself. Also, if you are trying to be healthier, it is useful to find a community that is such. We are part of the Crossfit Community. It is a group obsessed with health and fitness and therefore makes it easier to attain and maintain these things. Crossfit is about HIIT training, healthy food choices, alternative medicines, and overall creating a wellness lifestyle. There are other gyms that may share these principles, but they may be more difficult to locate as they are usually small and privately owned.

I do encourage you to find a health centered community; however, any of the aforementioned groups are still very beneficial. We all need to find/have our people of multiple interest groups. Fitness is not my only community. I have a very active and close family, I get involved coaching at the local high school, I have book clubs and community meetings. Your assignment this month is to start searching for yours, or appreciating the one you have by getting more involved.

Different stages of life will provide different community groups. Your interests and motivations will change throughout life. It is important to keep evolving. Family is one community that you will hopefully keep forever, but even that group will hopefully be growing and changing. Other things will change drastically. For example, Sororities and Fraternities are great college communities. Later in life that may be an Eagles Club or Kiwanis club. You will likely change homes and your neighborhood community will change. Friend groups will evolve. The important thing is to keep making new friends and new connections because you do not know who will be your next best friend. I have a best friend from undergrad and from graduate school. I met my recent best friend at a chamber of commerce meeting.

Keep in mind, there will be awkward beginning at times, you may find you dislike certain groups and that's OK. Keep experimenting until you find the groups that click. When you find your community, you will likely find you notice some of the following:

- Purpose in life

- More excitement to take on your day

- Looking forward to things

- Having more to life besides work

- Increased vitality

- Decreased depression

- More friends

Remember Maslow's hierarchy of needs? We spoke of this psychologist when discussing how loneliness creates inflammation. Community is another form of human connection that helps to satisfy that requirement. The total hierarchy is as follows:

Step 1 - Physiological-air, water, food, shelter, reproduction, sleep

Step 2 - Safety-employment, security, health, property, resources

Step 3 - Love and Belonging-friends, intimacy, family, sense of connection

Step 4 - Esteem-respect, self-esteem, status, recognition, freedom, strength

Step 5 - Self Actualization - the desire to be your best self

These are the stages of growth in human beings. If step one is not satisfied, you cannot reach 2. If you do not have 2 satisfied, you cannot skip to 4. If you want to reach step 5 and discover your true potential and attain the highest level of wellness, human connection and a sense of community is required.

Assignments

Try a HIIT gym or program

Get involved in Your community

Choose a Blood sugar plan (moderate fasting or adrenal fatigue)

Month 5

Detoxification, Slowing Down, and Getting Outdoors

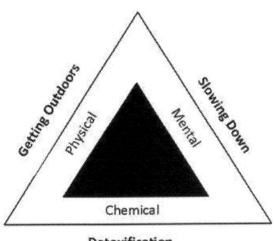

My Experience

I have done detox and refresh diet programs from multiple companies. I have had some great, some horrible, and some mediocre experiences. One of the main foods we will talk about in this chapter is dairy. As you heard in the introduction, this was the first food I eliminated back in undergraduate school. Eliminating dairy opened my eyes to the world of functional nutrition. I started to learn how to eat to make my body feel and perform better, not just eat for weight control. Although, I did lose weight by eliminating dairy.

The first program I bought into for detox was extremely supplement based. My gut could not handle all the products. I became miserably sick and had gas so bad I felt like I was being stabbed in the gut. I am not sharing this to scare you away from a detox. I just want you to be careful which supplements you choose. Also, diet and lifestyle are most important when detoxing. Do not get too dependent on products.

After fixing my digestive issues, I tried a different detox program and did awesome. I was already eating pretty clean beforehand from fixing my gut so I did not have any crazy revelations. I just made it through the detox without issue. I will be honest, not many detox protocols have ever provided much of a noticeable health difference for me. I would assume that is because my liver and gallbladder are one of the stronger attributes to my digestive system. My happy diet does consist of about 70% fat so I am pretty confident in its function. However, I have many friends and family that feel best on a detox type diet. Diets that stimulate detox or give the gallbladder a break usually look somewhat vegetarian/vegan. If you feel better on this type of diet, the detox life is likely a happy place for you at this moment. My sister lives on this type of program and it keeps her digestion optimal. It became necessary for her after two pregnancies, which we will discuss.

One detox protocol that I really did feel a benefit from was coffee enemas. I have attached the protocol in the appendix for this. I tried castor oil packs and gallbladder flushes, but coffee enemas made me feel amazing. They are great for an immune boost when you are struggling through back to back illnesses. They provide awesome mental clarity. They also provide a great deal of digestion relief. I highly encourage trying this during the detox month. Coffee enemas are used frequently in cancer therapy for their immune benefits. They particularly stimulate your liver and gallbladder detoxification systems. Let's delve into how and what detox entails.

Detox

The major detoxification reactions take place in the liver. Unfortunately, the lifestyles we live and world we live in can be very overbearing. Certain stresses in life make us need to take time to detox or give certain organs a break.

The predominant cause I consistently see that indicates a need for detox is an overload of hormones. This can happen from birth control, pregnancy, menopause, or other hormone therapies. Birth control can be particularly offensive. It has serious implications with artery health and heart disease. Did you know that most cases of stroke after an adjustment are in young females on Birth Control, not the older patient you would imagine? That is because of the clotting tendencies that happen with this drug. Birth control also depletes many B vitamins, increases yeast infections and clogs up the gallbladder creating discomfort in the upper abdomen. Birth control works by making you not have a full female cycle. Weather you bleed or not, birth control makes you not have a normal female cycle for however many months you are on it. It can take one month of detox for every year you were on the drug to restore a normal cycle. This can be very tricky for those expecting to get pregnant right after stopping the pill. You must be very friendly to you liver after stopping the pill if you wish to conceive. The Depo shot can cause infertility for up to ten years!

As a side note, there are many other ways to track your cycle to avoid getting pregnant besides drugs. Get a fertility tracker on your phone or buy one to put by your bedside and abstain on the days it says you are super fertile. Of course, it will take a few months after quitting the pill to even have a normal cycle to track so be aware of that. Now I digress.

A second reason that detox may be needed is a chronic cruddy diet. Although, I do not think I need to spend much time on this seems it is stressed in nearly every chapter.

Thirdly, if you have gallbladder attacks, this is the chapter for you! The liver and gallbladder are closely tied. Usually a problem in one does not come without the other. That is why many with a full gallbladder removal still have gallbladder attack symptoms. The problem was really in the liver. The liver creates the bile (that later sits in the gallbladder) to remove toxins and digest fats. The gallbladder is simply the storage unit. Now do you think the problem more likely in the storage unit or the organ filling the storage unit? A liver detox will usually provide great gall bladder relief.

If the detox protocol in the appendix is not enough to fully relieve an overburdened liver/gallbladder, other therapies may be added. That is why the coffee enema and castor oil packs are listed in the appendix. Bentonite clay can also be used as a detox supplement. You can use it as a drink or even turn it into a mud mask for your skin. The clay has amazing absorption properties and can draw excess toxins out of the skin or gut.

How Detox Works

Detox is done through the kidneys, skin, urine, sweat, or bile. The sweat carries out toxins during exercise. That can often contribute to the odor of the sweat. Many will notice less BO after detoxing. The sweat and urine can dispose of many water-soluble toxins. The more complex processes happen in the liver. Liver detox happens in three phases.

Phase 1 is an iron dependent phase that consists of oxidation, reduction, hydroxylation and sulfoxidation. This is a troublesome area for anemic patients that lack iron.

Phase 2 is a thyroid and glutathione dependent phase consisting of sulfation, glucuronidation, methylation and conjugation of amino acid. Most supplements focus on this area.

Phase 3 is metabolites being transferred to the gallbladder for removal. The gallbladder is fat consumption and thyroid hormone dependent. Hypothyroid patients often have insufficient detox.

So let's summarize. Detox requires a healthy thyroid hormone production, healthy fat consumption, adequate iron status (no anemia) and many diet related cofactors such as sulphur , methyl groups, and antioxidants. Note: methyl groups are usually attached to the B vitamins. It will look like "methylcobalamin" on a label, as an example. Also, those with MTHFR genetics problems will require help in this area.

So what can I do to detox?

A few things need to be addressed for detox help:

- Water Status
- Diet
- Slowing Down Life
- Getting rid of Toxic relationships
- Getting rid of toxic activities
- Utilizing the Help from Nature
- Sleep Hygiene
- Coffee Enema (See Appendix)
- Castor Oil Pack (See Appendix)

Water

Water is very needed for detox. It pushes toxins out the kidneys with urine and creates sweat. Dehydration is enough to inhibit some detoxification processes. Be sure to drink at least 8 glasses a day.

Slowing Down Life

It is important to note that excessive stress and workload affect the liver as much as toxins. Therefore, to treat the cause of liver dysfunction we must address these factors. This does not mean designing a meditation room and going full hippie. It simply means slowing down your life. Take a walk without any technological stimulus. Leave your phone off for a few hours. Enjoy your family and pets. Sit and drink coffee with loved ones. Have some quiet alone time. Go sit in a hammock in the sun. Usually nature is the best tool to slow down life.

Utilizing the Natural Help from Nature

Whether you like camping, hunting, hiking, walking the dog, or just having a cocktail on the porch you need to spend time outdoors. Nature has many stress relieving effects. Simply listening to nature sounds significantly changed perceived stress in one medical study. Time outside of man-made environment leads to reduced stress, improved mental function and improved mood. Simply being outside can relieve depression symptoms. As humans, we have built in evolutionary positive reactions to nature. After all, it is what our bodies were used to for thousands of years prior to the industrial revolution. Time in nature is slower, allows for rest, relaxation and recovery necessary to give our liver a break. This leads to one of the assignments this month; get outside daily and out of the city weekly. Go adventure in the woods.

Getting Rid of Toxic Relationships

I realize it can be odd to think of organs having an emotional tie. However, the examples are all around us. For example, do you ever have an acne break out from stress? Get a cold sore from stress? Lose weight from stress? If it can affect these things, why would it not affect the liver? In acupuncture, the liver is known to be related to the emotion of anger. Chronic anger leads to liver dysfunction in this discipline. This leads me to the topic of toxic relationships. If you are harboring anger toward a person, specifically your spouse, your liver will not function properly. This has implications on hormones, blood sugar, digestion and more. There are times where drastic action must be taken to either get therapy to heal a relationship, or to get rid of it!

Getting Rid of Toxic Activities

Do you have an activity which you just hate? Now, this can be anything from your job to volunteering at your kid's baseball. If an activity is making you miserable, not getting you toward an end goal, and wreaking havoc on your life then get rid of it. Quit feeling obligated to overbear yourself with senseless activities. Be selfish. Take on less unnecessary activities and obligations. If it is not getting you closer to your best life, why are you doing it? The only person capable of making you happy is you. Of course, you will have to do some things in life you do not want to, but hopefully that is to bring joy to your loved ones if not yourself. If nobody is benefiting though, ditch the activity or even the job. Now ditching a job may sound drastic. However, if your hours suck, you hate your coworker/ boss and your job is making you sick then you may need to quit. For example, many night shift jobs take years off your life due to the abnormality to your circadian rhythm (sleep cycle). You can grit and bear this fact, or find a healthier job!

Sleep Hygiene

Detox is a very powerful way to prevent or treat chronic illness. Normal detoxification happens at night. Acupuncture principles state that the time of day for best Liver and Gall Bladder activity are from 11PM until 3AM. If you are not sleeping during these hours, you are missing out on detox. Also, if you eat too late you will miss this phase. If your body is busy digesting, it will not be able to focus on detox. So over eating in the evening will affect this process.

Diet

You will find a complete food list in the appendix but let's discuss the purpose of these changes. We are trying to give the liver and gallbladder a rest. Many foods on the avoid list here are healthy foods; they just stress these organs too much. For example, the gall bladder helps with fat digestion. This program is low fat. The liver is involved in blood sugar control; therefore, we avoid high glycemic, processed foods. We also avoid caffeine because that stresses out the blood sugar by spiking adrenaline. The overall lesson in this protocol for this month is to eat as many vegetables as possible and keep your toxic load down. Be friendly to your body. Slow down. Quit the stimulants.

Dairy

As you can see from the appendix food list, one of the main food groups avoided in a detox food protocol is dairy. There are multiple reasons for dairy reactions. All 4 of these reasons will slow down liver detoxification. That is not to mention the high fat content of most dairy that can irritate those with a sluggish gallbladder.

1. Lactose Intolerance- Lactose is a sugar in milk. Many people lack the enzyme that digests milk and this creates severe gastric upset.

2. Casein allergy- this is the protein that would be tested for on an allergy panel. Casein is lowest in cheese, this is why many can handle cheese but not milk.

3. Overall Sugar intolerance-Just because you are not lactose intolerant due to an enzyme missing doesn't mean you won't react to lactose. Many just genetically do not digest sugar well or some have SIBO (small intestinal bacterial overgrowth) that makes them sugar intolerant.

4. High Histamine Food: On to genetics again, some people lack the enzyme necessary for histamine breakdown. There are foods that are high in histamine naturally. These increase allergy symptoms. Antihistamines are the medications used for allergies, make sense? Some people need to monitor histamine intake. Histamine is highest in fermented foods, particularly dairy products.

App recommendation: Food Intolerances is an app on your phone that looks like a strawberry. You can list suspected intolerances in here such as histamine and it will list all food containing the substance and rate the food on a low to high scale.

I know the milk conversation can get very heated. The dairy industry is one of the top performers in US agriculture. It's funny though, that milk producers are some of the only agriculture commercials in the US. You don't see commercials prodding you to eat a husk of corn each day. For some reason, the government and media want us to drink this substance. They are very disappointed that the almond industry is stealing their customers because people are getting smarter about their food choices. While I'm sure there are mostly financial motivations behind all this, let's see if we can find any nutritional explanation for drinking milk.

There are a multitude of reasons why dairy may be unfortunate for your diet. Even when you ignore the allergy/intolerance factors, it is high in calories and highly inflammatory. If you look at any food pyramid, regardless of philosophy dairy is a small triangle at the top of the pyramid. Many eat dairy as if it were the base of the triangle, it should not be the bulk of you meal. Instead, it should be a topping or garnish. Even with the keto diet, which is dairy friendly, portions must be controlled. Too much dairy can inhibit weight loss, and impair digestion. I would say dairy is the #1 cause of constipation in my office. In fact, constipation is sometimes a side effect of the keto diet and that is usually because people binge out on cheese.

So, what actually goes on when milk enters our systems? A typical response of our immune system when milk proteins are introduced is the release of mucus which blocks our throats and makes our voice raspy and hoarse, triggers ear infections and other flu-like symptoms which bother many kids regularly. You can observe this reaction rather quickly. If you give your child a bowl of ice cream and within the next hour they start having a runny nose and itchy face, they are having a reaction to the dairy. Not to mention some of the other sugar effects like an overly emotional, un-rational child. A few other things we tend to observe on kids is dark circles under the eyes and a white line across the nose. The dark circles are from chronic histamine release overloading the liver and the white lines are from constant itching.

The Hormone Problem

While no hormone inside milk is actually beneficial for our health, there is one hormone in particular you should pay attention to and this is the Insulin-like Growth Factor (IGF-1). Humans tend to produce this hormone during their adolescence and it's not healthy when it's too much. Additionally, so-called fitness and health shops will sell this IGF-1 hormone as steroid drug or supplement to enhance muscle mass in humans or animals. Yep, that substance is actually an anabolic steroid and it's administered to both humans and animals to help them bulk up. Therefore, consider this when your kids are drinking cow milk as they are actually taking amounts of the IGF-1 as well, from the cows that make the milk. IGF-1 is one example of the Obesegens contained in milk. These compounds, I'm sure you guessed from the name, increase obesity regardless of calorie content. There are multiple hormones in milk that have this affect. In another obesegen story, rats that were fed antibiotic treated food vs. not became obese; same calorie content, just different quality. Think about it, do you really think lack of physical activity is the only cause for the obesity spike in this country? No! Our food quality has changed due to these obesegens.

The hormones are actually a triggering factor of cancer as well. More specifically, medical researchers have found out that IGF-1 is a key factor in the development of colon, breast, and prostate cancers. According to a report published on the late 90s in Science magazine, males that show high levels of IGF-1 hormone have a 4x increased risk to grow full-escalated prostate cancer compared to males with lower levels of IGF-1.

Casein Protein and Fat

Some of you may wonder at this point about the so-called "low fat" milk versions. Low fat also means added sugar. When we lose the fatty flavor, we have to add something else in. Most skim milk contains 10g of sugar per glass, so if you drink 2 glasses a day, you could have just had a chocolate bar.

The main protein in milk is Casein. Casein is a vivid allergen compound which triggers the buildup of mucus in the system. As we all realize, mucus is directly occurring in flu and flu-like symptoms. Therefore, if you suffer from these problems, you better avoid eating any dairy as these will make the issue of mucus worse. This also affects your bowels. Casein makes some people have very runny stool due to the mucous production. Of course, other components in milk can warrant the opposite effect. I find dairy to be the #1 cause of constipation or diarrhea in my office, it just depends which component you react to and gut bacteria present.

The Calcium Myth

We've been told as kids that our milk is intended to make our bones harder and stronger, right? From a theoretical perspective, this has a point but in reality, this isn't as accurate as it seems. The issue is that calcium in milk cannot be utilized as it is, because it requires levels of phosphorus and magnesium to be absorbed by the system.

Calcium is a vital nutrient for sure. The most ideal and healthy sources of calcium naturally occur in dark green leafy veggies like kale and spinach. And this is perfectly reasonable as cows themselves get their calcium from grass, which is a leafy green as well.

Milk and Acne

A man named Jerome K. Fisher carried out a study lasting 10 years and examining over 1000 teens suffering from acne. In his study published in American Dermatological Association, milk was found to be the main factor that contributed to the onset of acne in some of the teenagers. He noted that dairy is loaded with fats and milk sugars, and can make acne problems worse. Additionally, he supported that excess amounts of hormones being released by a pregnant cow could convert into androgens. Androgens, as a result, put the sebaceous glands that produce oil in our pores into an overload and this eventually clogs pores and causes acne. Acne basically appears when these pores are clogged. Androgens in excess can also inhibit or slow down liver detoxification.

Milk, Allergies, and Ear Infections

Based on study findings of the Academy of Allergy, Asthma, and Immunology, cow's milk is the leading culprit of food allergies in kids. Many researchers have also linked milk with the onset of respiratory infections including ear problems and asthma. Doctors note this on a frequent basis, when examining children. Dr. Oski says that he suggest to parents with children suffering from these infections to reduce and avoid dairy as the only solution to improve their symptoms. Within just a few weeks of cutting down dairy, the kids are no longer bothered by these issues and no longer rely on antibiotics and pills to control they symptoms. Often a complete elimination is needed to see a change/ elimination in symptoms. This also has implications with older children that wet the bed at night. This has been highly correlated with uncontrolled allergies and their effect on the adrenals and Aldosterone hormone (anti-peeing hormone).

Milk, Colic and Gas

It may be surprising, but even a baby doesn't drink milk directly, he may take it from its mother who drinks it. A study published on the American Dietetic Association Journal, who examined 272 breastfeeding mothers, has found that mothers who ate certain types of foods such as cow's milk, had babies affected more by colics

Now concerning the issue of gas, Hippocrates was probably the first physician to notice a connection between milk and gas, years ago. It is also speculated that in the U.S alone, 30 million people suffer from lactose intolerance, which shows up in symptoms like bloating, gas, diarrhea, and rashes. If this looks familiar to you, try quitting milk and dairy for just two weeks and note down the benefits.

Milk Substitutes

It can be very confusing to shop for dairy alternatives because almost all of them have some kind of negative connotation to them. With almond milk, there is not much protein or nutritional content. With soy, there is the estrogenic concern. With coconut, its fat content scares some. So what do we do? My philosophy with most things is the find the least of the evils. For example, coconut cream is fatty, but it has less of an effect on my sinus and gut than heavy dairy cream would so I put coconut cream in my coffee. The extra fat actually lessens the acidity of the coffee and provides my brain with energy besides just caffeine. I quit eating cereal but if I need to drizzle milk on something or I am cooking pancakes, I use almond milk. I buy the unsweetened kind so that I do not spike my blood sugar and try to buy brands with the least amount of ingredients on the label.

The more ingredients mean the more dangerous additives like carrageenan. Almond milk should be mostly almonds and water. If I want cheese, I do buy the tofu derived cream cheese or possibly nut cheeses. There are a few brands that taste decent and most of the reasons you need cream cheese or sour cream is for cooking so these alternative options are not noticeably different from the original milk versions.

Also, as stated before, when you do eat dairy it should be a topping not a main course. Better to only stimulate the immune response occasionally and in small doses. Also, if you do buy dairy, please buy the organic or grass fed versions. Grass fed butter and ghee can be OK to use. Butter has very little dairy protein or lactose as it is mostly fat. Therefore, it does not trigger much of the immune response.

Assignments

Eliminate Dairy and follow the detox dietary list

Detox one activity from your life to allow your schedule to slow down

Get Outdoors Daily, Away From the City Weekly

Month 6

Light Therapy, Paleo Lifestyle, and Posture

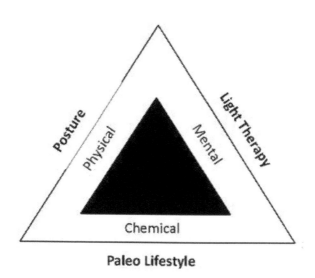

Paleo Lifestyle

My Experience

I am a firm believer in practice what you preach. I have done every protocol described in this book. I will say though, my journey into a health/wellness lifestyle and career started with Paleo. As stated in the introduction, I found Paleo when I started Crossfit. I soon discovered the infinite potential our diet has on affecting our energy, pain, and overall well being. When I committed to Paleo, my muscle pains decreased exponentially especially after hard workouts. I was no longer falling asleep during class. I accomplished more per day. I got better at my sport. I had a higher capacity for work. I also lost a lot of fat mass, approximately 6%, and all without calorie counting. I was actually eating a ton! Of course, part of my calorie intake was to keep up with a somewhat excessive amount of training I was doing at the time. Point being, when I started Crossfit, I was miserably sore and could barely handle the work load because my diet sucked. I remember one day having pasta at Olive Garden. It was a "healthy well rounded meal" if you look at the Standard American Diet (SAD Diet). I was so sore I could barely do a simple rowing workout the next day.

Fast forward to now. I definitely still fall off the bandwagon as most people do sometimes. Even when I do though, it is nice to know that the reason I feel cruddy is because I veered from my happy diet. You will find your own happy diet while working through this book. Mine is a Keto/Paleo mix that basically concentrates on low sugar and carbs. I can handle a little cheese and butter but besides that Paleo is my way to go. Everyone will be different, but Paleo is my go-to for a healthy long term eating plan.

What is Paleo?

Paleo is the hunter/gatherer diet that we humans are evolutionarily programmed to eat. This consists of high protein, plant fiber, and fat as well as high activity level. Our ancestors could not run to Walmart and buy fruit or cookies as we do now, sugar containing food was a rarity. Hunter/gatherers ate mostly what they could find in the wild. This means game meat/fish, root vegetables, fruit when in season, and maybe low amounts of nuts or grains when found. Those are the basics of a paleo diet. For a simple paleo shopping list, stick to my five food rule:

1. Meat/Fish
2. Vegetable
3. Fruit
4. Sweet potato
5. Coconut products

History Fun facts

Other hunter gatherer societies still existing today do not know the health disparities we do in the United States. They have no "metabolic syndromes" suggesting that what we have been taught about nutrition is likely false. Even cavities started showing up in the fossil record only shortly after humans started farming grains. The Primal Man actually lived longer than our civilized ancestors (60's average by fossil record). Our current life expectancy in the US is in the 70's and dropping. Many developed countries are still only in the 60's range for life expectancy. Our caveman ancestors also died mostly in accidents/age and not disease.

Food Pyramid Upside Down

"Americans will always do the right thing---AFTER they have exhausted all the wrong options."-Winston Churchill

If you have not heard what I am saying yet, I will say it again. We have been lied to about what a healthy diet contains. Our health information in this country is OWNED by corporations. It is not put out by the government for the greater educational good; it is lining someone's pockets. Once you understand that, it will make sense why everything you were previously taught is false. I want you to turn your previous nutritional education upside down quite literally. Take that stupid carbohydrate heavy, diabetes stimulating, heart disease producing food pyramid and flip it upside down. To be healthy, we essentially need to do the opposite of what is popular or promoted.

I have created a new pyramid for you. I think this is the most accurate way to approach your food groups. This will keep a very nutrient rich variety of vitamins and minerals in your life while still addressing protein adequately. I will say the pyramid flipped to having meat on the bottom is still accurate because protein has more calories that salad. However, the picture below is a better picture for cup size quantity servings. Notice, the most cups is of water eh? The below pyramid would translate to 8 cups of water, 4-6 of vegetables, 3-4 of proteins, 1-2 of fruits, 1 of nuts and spices as needed.

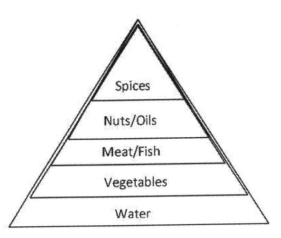

The Wrong Options

The best thing to do is avoid the middle isles at the grocery store. Shop the perimeter of the grocery store and you will avoid most of the offensive foods. Do not buy boxed food, freezer meals, and most canned products. If you have to read a label, skip it. Few stores do have a health food section, if a food is truly healthy it will have a short ingredient list. It will be in English, not chemistry words. An example: Paleo mayonnaise is made with Avocado Oil, Organic Eggs, Organic Egg Yolks, Organic Vinegar, Sea Salt, and Organic Rosemary Extract. Miracle Whip is made from water, soybean oil, high-fructose corn syrup, vinegar, modified corn starch, eggs, salt, natural flavor, mustard flour, potassium sorbate, paprika, spices, and dried garlic. Which do you think is healthier? The one with high fructose corn syrup and whatever ambiguous ingredients fall beneath "natural flavors" or the one made from primarily avocado?

We will discuss the eliminated foods list and why each item is offensive. First, here is a list of some food groups we avoid with Paleo:

Grains

Dairy

Legumes

Processed Food

Alcohol

Starch

Sugars*

*PALEO Treats

Do not overdose on "paleo" sweets. Just because they are made with natural ingredients and less offensive sugars, does not mean they're a freebie. They are still affecting insulin. They will inhibit weight loss. They need to be viewed as the treat that they are and be eaten in moderation. If you go Paleo and still eat 3 servings of fruit a day, honey in your tea and paleo brownies, you will not get the full benefit of the lifestyle and you will still corrupt your insulin sensitivity. That being said, Maple syrup is by far the least offensive sweetener if you need dessert.

Where are the carbs?

Many are under the misconception that Paleo is a no-carbohydrate diet. That is not the case. We just have to redefine carbohydrates. Many think of carbohydrates as only grains or desserts. However, fruits, vegetables and root vegetables are also carbohydrates. The carbohydrates allowed in this program are low glycemic fruit, sweet potatoes, and other root vegetables. It is important to remember that all starches spike blood sugar. Use sparingly, they all promote fat storage. The government recommended whole grains are not necessary. Grains all create inflammation and are unnaturally processed. They also promote fat storage. However, the least offensive grains if you "need them" are wild rice, quinoa, Ezekiel bread, or gluten free oats.

Why not Dairy?

There are some that embrace a variation called lacto-paleo, meaning they eat dairy. I have provided an extended explanation for dairy in previous chapters but here is a short synopsis. Most conventional (regular store bought) dairy is contaminated with loads of antibiotics, hormones, and chemicals. Dairy increases histamine, phlegm, and allergies. Most yogurts, creamers, and low fat products spike blood sugar and hence increase inflammation. Remember, skim milk has sugar is added to replace flavor from fat removal. This is true for all "low fat" dairy.

If you do consume dairy, buy raw, organic, and full fat. Dairy is the most important product to buy organic at the grocery store.

Why no legumes?

Legumes contain lectins that inflame your gut and cause intestinal discomfort. In short, lectins give you gas. Hence, the beans bean they are good for your heart but the more you eat the more you fart rhyme. They also often have a high glycemic index so do not help control blood sugar. Legumes include peanuts, beans, chickpeas, and peas.

Foods to Include

Healthy Fat: Good sources of healthy fat are olive oil, coconut oil, ghee, animal fat for cooking, fish oil supplement, nut oils, and avocado. AVOID canola, sunflower, vegetable, margarine, safflower, and shortening. Many of these oils are man-made and not recognized by our digestive system or are processed improperly. Even olive oil can be tampered with. Be sure your olive oil is not split with canola to make it cheaper.

Protein: Simply speaking, this is everything with fins, feathers, feet or eggs. I will tell you too that quality matters. How an animal is raised affects the nutrient content of the meat. If you eat an obese cow, you are more likely to be obese right? Therefore, it is best to look for words like free range, grass fed, and organic. These animals (or their eggs) will have higher quality of fat and micronutrients. When buying fish look for wild caught for the same reason, the omega 3 will be higher in wild fish than those raised in a pool (farm raised). Some examples of protein are beef, chicken, turkey, lamb, duck, and eggs. There is also free roaming game such as venison, bison, or elk. The wild game tend to have the lowest fat content.

Veggies

Eat as much as possible and as many colors as possible. Every color of vegetable signifies a different nutrient content. For example, orange foods like carrots have more Vitamin A. Deep greens and purples are higher in antioxidants. Reds help blood flow and nitric oxide pathways that can prevent clots and stroke. Reds may also help with menstrual disorders or pain due to this blood stimulating effect as well. There is one category of plants called nightshades. These can be troublesome for the auto-immune patient. They include potatoes, peppers, eggplants, and tomatoes. These patients I suggest follow the leaky gut chapter to address this group. For most individuals, nightshades are still healthy.

Moderate fruit

You will want to stick to low glycemic fruits. There is a full list in the appendix, but berries tend to be safest. When buying organic vs. not, look into the clean 15 and dirty dozen. The clean 15 are avocados, sweet corn, pineapples, cabbage, onions, sweet peas frozen, papayas, asparagus, mangos, eggplant, honeydew melon, kiwi, cantaloupe, cauliflower, and broccoli. The dirty dozen are strawberries, spinach, nectarines, apples, grapes, peaches, cherries, pears, tomatoes, celery, potatoes and sweet bell peppers. My rule of thumb is that if you eat the peel buy organic, if not, conventional is fine. This will keep your pesticide exposure to a minimum.

Nuts and Seeds

These foods are high fat and high protein which is their blessing as well as their curse. They are very nutrient dense. They are great in small doses but detrimental in large doses due to calorie content and lectin content.

The outer coating of nuts can really irritate the gut lining and ileo-cecal valve if taken in large amounts. Try to stick to raw or soaked nuts or nut butters to decrease the gut irritating effect. Remember: many paleo baked goods are made with almond flour. Do not overdose on this or you will be hurting.

Spices and Herbs

These are how you make your food taste good. When getting away from sugary sauces, many find food bland. This means more experimentation with spices and oils. A trick I learned from my mentor is if it smells good together. It tastes good together.

Do not skimp on the spices. Many even have healing qualities. For example, turmeric is commonly used for controlling inflammation.

The 80% Rule (or 80/20 rule)

"Perfection is impossible. However, striving for perfection is not. Do the best you can under the conditions that exist. That's what counts." -John Wooden

One last point I would like to mention with this program is that 100% perfect is not necessary. You will make mistakes. We have discussed this before. Do not give up just because you had one pizza night. Keep moving forward. Know that 80% perfect and 20% imperfect is adequate for a maintenance program. As I have mentioned, it is great to have months where you really grind it out for 30 days and see how well you can do, but most people do not last beyond the 30 days if they expect 100 % perfection 100% of the time. If you want to make more than 30 days of progress on your body, accept that you will have drawbacks, just like in every other aspect of life. Having 100% good days in life that would be great, but not really realistic right?

Take Home (Food Related) Points

❏ Eat as many vegetables as possible every day

❏ Eliminate as many processed foods as possible-avoid premade/fast food

❏ Limit carbohydrates, especially those containing sugar

❏ Include a healthy fat in every meal

❏ Include protein each meal, especially for breakfast

❏ Buy organic when possible

❏ Drink water

❏ 80/20 rule

Get Outdoors or Get Light Therapy

Paleo lifestyle also consists of ample outdoor time in order to get energy from the sun. Sunlight is a nutrient. It is a nutrient all life depends on. Sunlight in humans is known as an activator of vitamin D. Vitamin D has innumerous actions in the body but most are involved in boosting immunity and utilization of calcium.

Let's not forget sunlight's impact on mood. Sunlight has direct correlation with Serotonin. Heard of seasonal depression? It basically means less sunlight equals less serotonin. You can boost serotonin with diet and exercise. This basically comes down to balancing blood sugar as previously suggested. I am a firm believer though that sunlight can never be replaced. Even look at your pets. They are more energetic on sunny days. They bask in the light of the window. All creatures crave the light and function more happily and energetically with it.

In the non-freezing times of year it is best to get at least 15 minutes of no sunscreen sunlight. Even if you can push it with a few t shirt minutes during the spring or fall that is best. Now, for people like us Michiganders living in the Up North, we may need to supplement our light spectrum needs. Sounds interesting eh? Taking light as a supplement? This is what I am suggesting though. There are many types of light therapy but a great full spectrum therapy is infrared saunas. We also use therapeutic laser in our office. I highly recommend using saunas like this if you do not have the stamina to go outside shirtless in winter. We cannot all be my husband. He is a ginger, which means he utilizes Vit D more efficiently than other skin tones. He is also a total psycho and will run around shirtless in the snow and even jump in the lake if it's not covered in ice. If this doesn't sound like you, find an infrared sauna.

Infrared saunas are a type of sauna that uses heat and light to help relax and detoxify the body. They are known to have anti-aging effects, increased detoxification, pain reduction, joint and muscle support, and cardiovascular healing. They're also believed to have a stress management effect.

How Infrared Saunas Work

Light therapies can have an inflammation-lowering effect, can act as an antioxidant nutrient, can activate the cells, can help with wound healing, can boost metabolism and can help remove toxins from the body. All these aspects you should be getting from the sun. Organisms, such as us, have physiology that is very dependent on light. Think this is all bogus? Put a plant in a dark room for the entire winter and see if it survives.

Most light therapy works by inserting photons. Photons are absorbed by the bonds in the body's molecules, and water and mitochondrial activity are changed in the cell. Many chiropractors offer laser therapies that do this as well.

Other Benefits of Light (Sun or Alternatives)

Light helps reduce chronic pain including arthritis. Many recognize that when they are in a warm environment that hurt less. This is why the baby boomers all move to Florida or Arizona. Both places have more sunlight so you feel less pain. Chronic Pain is regulated by Serotonin. Sunlight increases this causing less pain. That is why most pain is worst in the darker winter months. Depressed individuals often experience more pain because of this mechanism.

Go Primal Posture!

I call it the Paleo Lifestyle, not the Paleo Diet right? That is because it requires more than just food changes to reach its full potential. We discussed outdoor time and sunlight requirements. The other part of this lifestyle is moving, lifting, walking, sprinting, or interval training daily. **Nearly all chronic diseases are related to lack of or decrease in movement.**

Most of this has been discussed at length in earlier chapters. This chapter I want to delve into posture. Our chronic lack of movement has destroyed our posture. Something as simple as rolled forward shoulders can impair breathing and cause asthma. Every inch your head goes forward from your shoulders adds a bowling ball size weight to your head. 80% of headaches and neck pain are due to the position in your posture. Very small differences in posture have a huge impact on our health. So simply by reverting back to our primal postures, we can prevent some disease and discomfort.

Posture and Breathing

Based on late research findings, poor posture can be incredibly destructive to healthy and essential breathing patterns. You really don't need a scientist or doctor to make this connection, you can try it directly yourself.

Bend over as if you are trying to make your knees touch the breast area. Once you there in this position, start to breathe deeply. Is this challenging? If your posture is misaligned even a bit, it can affect your ease of breathing as it interferes' with diaphragm function. Now pin your shoulders back against your chair. Breathing should automatically get way easier due to proper alignment of the diaphragm.

We see that the diaphragm is responsible for extending our lungs so we can receive the largest amount of air and oxygen from outside into our systems. When the diaphragm pulls down, it allows the lungs and the chest cavity to enlarge so that the air circulates through. When the diaphragm is in relaxation mode, the lungs and the chest relax too and push air out.

Diaphragm activation affects organ position, digestion, oxygen capacity, relaxation response, neck posture, Mid Back posture, sinus pressure, detoxification and more. It is the major pump for non-arterial fluids.

Did you know that we breathe on average 25, 000 times a day? If your diaphragm is blocked (as a result of bad posture), you will not be able to breathe deeply. This of course results in your cells getting less amounts of oxygen. As we mentioned earlier, cells that don't get sufficient amounts of oxygen can't function at their best. Thus, the connection here is pretty evident. Great posture translates to a great functioning diaphragm and ultimately overall body cells.

Posture and Emotion

Bad posture isn't only equal to body pain. It can also affect your mood. Here is an example--picture someone that is depressed and anxious and what their body posture looks like. Do his shoulders and head pop-up confidently and project toward the front? Or does he look the opposite. 90% of the time, his body has a shrunk, slumped over posture. Posture respectively affects his mood and vice versa. Here is why this happens. Our brains store the majority of our physical control movements and our emotional reactions together. Our feelings and emotions specifically are stored in the part of our brain called "the limbic system" (or the emotional brain). The manner we carry our bodies has a clear impact on our emotional brains (the limbic system). That is why "power postures" exists. When you puff up your chest and bring your shoulders back and stand up straight, you are automatically more confident and seen as so by your peers.

Creating Good Posture

Good posture means symmetry. It means equal weight on both legs. It means front to back and side to side balance. Good posture is the muscles on the body all working in equilibrium. Some of this is done by conscious control with muscle training and other parts are subconscious. For example, you do not tell your body to breath, but you can control the cadence. It is the same with most postural muscles, they work whether you tell them to or not. However, when trying to correct posture, you will have to do some active muscle exercise or tell your muscle where proper position lies.

Correcting posture is most effective with a combination of chiropractic adjustments to free spinal segments while neurologically activating muscles and adding exercises to retrain these muscles and strengthen them. This is best done with Physical Therapy. A PT (physical therapist) will know when you are creating imbalances with certain exercises and correct you. There are also specific techniques for core activation and diaphragm function in this field. One technique called DNS (dynamic neuromuscular stabilization) is very effective at correcting posture by activation of core muscles and proper breathing.

The most effective exercise to correct posture is called "Paleo Chair," "Yoga Squat," and many other things. The easiest way to see this though is in young kids. Toddlers often have perfect posture (until they get ruined by technology). If you watch them sit in the bottom position of a squat it is perfect. The knees are over the ankles, the shoulders are upright and not rolled, their neck has a perfect curve, etc. Your goal should be to achieve this position and I guarantee you will have great posture. It is the perfect combination of muscle training. I suggest when starting to not go full depth and to hang onto something until you are strong enough to go hands free. If you can go hands free, try graduating to being able to hold your arms up next to your ears.

Here are many activities that can help improve posture:

- Perform balance exercises to assist your joints in their new structure. Pilates, Yoga, Tai Chi and pretty much anything on a balance ball/pad.

- Engage in weight lifting activities that engage the back muscles like rowing, pull ups, deadlifts, Lat pull downs, and any kind of barbell squat.

- Adopt functional exercises into your workouts. Remember, these are exercises that mimic activities you do in daily life.

- Your posture muscles are big strong ones. They require weighted training to fully correct. Keep in mind, things like yoga can be "weights" because you are holding your body weight in difficult positions. The Yoga Squat mentioned earlier is a good start but you will become proficient at this posture faster if you do full workout classes.

- Practice proper breathing for 15 min or more a day. That can be during yoga/meditation.

- Be sure to check your work ergonomics. In short, this means keeping good posture in your workplace.

Ergonomics

Ergonomics is the practice of designing your workplace to suit your body and your needs. In my life, I pay attention to table height to keep my back happy. I buy hand tools to prevent carpal tunnel and wrist injury. I elevate my computer to write notes so that I do not crane my neck. I have a balance ball stool for when I sit. These are all ways that I design my workplace to keep me healthy. I also make sure that I practice proper lifting and body mechanics while I work to prevent injury.

It is movement we do repetitively each day that affect our overall function. Be sure that the position you stand, sit, or lift every day is not creating bad habits or bad health. Either purchase the tools to alleviate your issues or make a presentation to your boss why you need a standing desk, new chair, etc.

Another overlooked part of ergonomics is movement. Get your steps in! Sitting is the new smoking. Get up and move around if you have a sedentary job and it will help your overall health.

My experience:

A few months into doing Crossfit people started to mistake me for a gymnast. I did not think I had poor posture before, but exercise made me hold myself differently. I would ask if it had to do with my height and they consistently said "No, It's your posture." Now I had always been an athlete and had never had this accusation. I know it was sheerly due to the training with functional movements and chiropractic care. A functional movement means a weight bearing exercise that would translate into daily life. For example, we squat all day every day to sit up from couches, chairs, cars, toilets etc. Deadlifts would be what we use to pick up and move a box or furniture. A push up is what would help us get off the floor if we fell down. You use a pull up to get you out of the water after swimming in the pool. See what I am saying? These kinds of movements are what correct posture and they are not used in every gym setting.

I know I have talked about Chiropractic a bit already, but we truly are the posture doctors. We mobilize the spine to allow movement into proper posture. We free the diaphragm for proper breathing. We coach on proper biomechanics for exercise. We give suggestions on proper workplace ergonomics. The list goes on. If you are having trouble forcing yourself into good posture, chances are a proper adjustment will get you the rest of the way there.

Assignments

Embrace a Paleo Dietary Lifestyle

Evaluate your posture at work every day-be sure to have posture friendly ergonomics

Get Real Sunlight for 20 min a day or Try a Light Therapy Alternative in Winter.

Month 7

Yoga, Functional Medicine, and Meditation

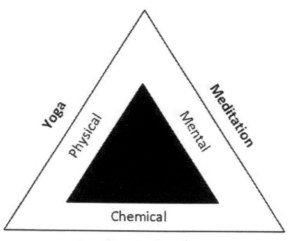

Functional Medicine

My Experience

Functional Medicine was one technique that changed my health when I started seeing Dr. Huff. I talked in earlier chapters how it helped heal my gut and blood sugar problems. It is a practice that teaches you about your own body and how to keep it functioning at 100%.

Functional Medicine also taught me to be friendly to my adrenal glands. My doctor knew at the first visit that I was an adrenaline junkie, looking for the next challenge and risk at all times. I never settled down. I went from grad school to Crossfit to intense outdoor sports without any relaxing activities. He suggested that I find other sports, since there was no way I could quit working out, that are less adrenaline pushers. I decided to take some time for yoga.

The first time I did yoga, I thought it was just glorified stretching mixed with some funny noises. What I found was a class that challenged me mentally and physically. There were different limits to be pushed than in a typical workout. It was at the moment where I was upside down with my feet climbing up a wall that I decided it was kind of fun too. Yoga added a whole new element to my fitness. It allowed to me squat deeper, move better, and hit my core greater than any other exercise. Overall, yoga just made me feel more stable.

Yoga also introduced me to meditation. I learned how much energy a few minutes of silence can give you. In a world of overstimulation, just 5-10 minutes of quiet thought can make a world of difference.

Meditation

Meditation looks different for everyone. Adding this relaxation technique to your life does not mean that you have to buy a tie dye rug, listen to flutes playing, and smoke green. My definition of meditation is finding time in your life for some peace and quiet to simply breathe and let the brain take a break. Most people will find that when they do this they actually find the answers to more of their problems because their brain has time to thoroughly consider them. That is why napping does not count as meditation. Although 20 minute naps mid-day do have their advantages.

Have you ever laid awake at night, your brain just going like crazy, thinking about all your dilemmas and trying to fix them to a point where sleeping is impossible? This generally occurs because either your circadian rhythm is whack or you just never allow your brain the time to wander in silence at any other point during the day. If you feel that you need a notepad on your nightstand to get your thoughts down while you are lying in bed, then you are in desperate need of meditation time earlier in your day. You need time to settle down to sleep at night; it is not the time to solve the world's problems. Pick a different slotted time in the day for that.

Meditation for me means sitting with my dog in the morning with coffee alone and in silence or walking the dog down a trail in silence. Basically, I require my dog for proper meditation time. However, my husband has a ritual where he lies in the dark basement gym before bed and stretches for 20 minutes. We also recently purchased a guided meditation unit that incorporates sound and light. It is called a Kasina unit from Mind Place. This is a great way to pick pre-programmed sessions all toward different purposes. For example, you would choose an awaken session for the morning or a relaxation one when feeling overwhelmed. Of course these units can be expensive so if you cannot use it at a doctor's office, it may be a bit of an investment to get at home. If you don't want to buy into meditation technology, do it the old fashion way and you will still get great results.

Find your own optimal meditation technique and atmosphere. For many men I would argue that sitting in a deer stand in the freezing cold morning is actually a form of mediation. It is a time to turn the brain off from constant stimulation of society and relax. Your meditation strategy should change based on your goals. If I want a complete brain shut off I do puzzles. If I need to brainstorm a problem, I walk. If I need to blow off stress I do deep breathing in the dark in the massage room at our office. Moral of the story is to find the activities that help you cope with stress the best. I mean, if I hit a certain level of anger, no meditation will do. I have to go throw some weights around the gym. Intense exercise is often the only way I can get rid of anxiousness and tension. Find your method. Do not just hold things in and push them out of your consciousness. That just leads to more problems.

Positive Affirmations

Positive affirmations are a great way to get into meditation. This can be really helpful to those feeling lost, self-conscious, or anxiety ridden. A technique I learned once was to go through the following affirmations to sequentially satisfy the different layers of your brain in order to reach a meditative state.

I am safe

I am loved

I am cared for

I am infinite

I am safe

In this affirmation you are to think of all the ways that your basic needs have been met. Think about your shelter, food, water, etc. Knowing your basic needs are met is one way to relax your brain and bring attention to the fact that you are OK. There is no dire threat to your existence so you can relax.

I am loved

As said in earlier chapters, community is very important to the human brain. A feeling of love and belonging is needed for optimal survival. We need to not only think of loving intimate relations here. Think about family, spouse, friends, teams, church, pets, etc.

I am cared for

This is slightly different than the loved affirmation. Cared for should means someone is keeping you alive a safe. This may mean your job or your boss and coworkers. This may mean your parents and family helping you out. This may be your spouse caring for you while you are ill. This is when you think of all the people you are thankful for that help you along in life.

I am infinite

The previous three topics should have relaxed your brain enough to get into some serious down time. I am infinite is where you can really wander. Think about who you are or want to become. Tell yourself you will reach your goals and plot a way to get to them. This is time for true discovery.

These affirmations are a great meditation technique. You may also use this anytime that anxiety and fear are overpowering you. If you are prone to anxiety attacks and feel one approaching, find a quiet place immediately and start saying these "I am "assertions repeatedly in sequence. Don't forget to breathe! Lack of oxygen makes anxiety worse and many of us hold our breath when stressed and frustrated.

Stress Reflex Vessels

Another tip during mediation, especially for anxiety/stress, is to place your hands on you temples. There is a blood vessel that travels just above the lateral eyebrow up to your hairline. This is a natural stress reflex (called a neurovascular in Applied Kinesiology). When we are stressed, we almost all naturally grab out forehead. That is because pressure on this vessel helps regulate pressure in the head. Thus it helps us settle from stressful situations. So I recommend light pressure be held to these vessels when you feel like you are about to lose it. If you can feel for a pulse (it's there but very light) hold it until both sides slow and get into unison.

Yoga

Probably the easiest way to engage in meditation each day is by joining a yoga gym. Not only do most yoga facilities offer meditation specific classes but yoga in itself is quite Zen. You even have a chill time to lay there at the end of each class called shavasana. There are many different yoga techniques and styles. Each class is designed for different results. For example, a vinyasa class is usually where you get the best workout. Yin classes are slower stretching.

Yin Vs Yang Exercise

Everything in Chinese medicine and yoga focuses on the two sides of nature, Yin and Yong. They are based on the principle that everything in nature is in balance by an opposite: Cold or Hot, Good or Evil, Up or Down, Girl or Boy, Dark or Light. Yin is female, cold and dark. Yang is male, hot and light. Yin is to create outward movement and yang is to create inward. These energies are supposed to be in balance to create optimal health. When you get too much yang, you can become yin deficient, manifesting as certain disorders and vice versa.

It is important that we think of exercise in yin and yang as well. Most of us focus too much on yang exercise. We love the pain, the burn, the adrenaline. We feel like in order to gain a benefit from an exercise it has to be this intense calorie burn. However, both sides of exercise are necessary and feed different systems of health (yin or yang). Most yoga falls into the yin category of exercise. It is slow, deep stretching, and does not heat the body up much accept or a few classes such as Vinyasa or Buti yoga. Tai chi is yin. Most other typical exercise I can think of is yang.

We need balance. The Yin exercise junkie is your typical yogie. However, if they do not do any yang they tend to be under-muscled and have low cardiovascular endurance. On the flip side the yang exercise junkie is likely to get burned out adrenals or injured due to lack of yin. I see both in my office. Usually therapy for the yogie is to lift more and the crossfitter (all yang) is to stretch more. When yogis try to stretch more due to injury, they often get weaker and worse off because they are becoming more yin, which they already are. I hope this is starting to make sense. NEITHER ATHLETE WILL REACH FULL RECOVERY OF THEY DO NOT ENGAGE IN THE OPPOSITE SIDE OF FITNESS. As a chiropractor, both are hard to treat of they do not change their exercise routine. The super yogie vegan is the hardest to get better due to extreme lack in muscle mass to support their joints. When they come to me, it is usually due to muscle weakness complaints that do not get better without steak and weights. The overstretched muscle is the most difficult to heal. Be sure not to misunderstand me here. Stretching is still very important for the nutrition and health of a joint. Just do not take it too far.

What Is The Importance Of Maintaining Flexibility

There are many reasons why having a flexible body is essential to your health and well-being. Flexibility can be termed as the ability of your joints and body parts to execute their full range of motion. Flexibility is needed to perform every day activities with relative ease. To get out of bed, raise children, or sweep the floor, we need flexibility. Flexibility tends to deteriorate with age, often due to a sedentary lifestyle and not arthritis as many tend to believe. Without adequate flexibility, daily activities become more challenging to perform. Over time, we create body movements and posture habits that can lead to reduced mobility of joints and compromised body positions. The lazy boy chair is probably the worst thing to happen to the elderly spine because it keeps the spine in a misaligned position for hours on end. Airplane seats are probably the only worse position. They both reverse the normal curve of the low back. Staying active and stretching regularly help prevent this loss of mobility, which ensures independence as we age. Being flexible significantly reduces the chance of experiencing back pain. It also extremely reduces the risk of falls and other injuries.

The Benefits of Flexibility

There are some ways to test your flexibility. One of the most common ways, according to fitness experts, is to check if you can touch your toes while standing up with both legs straight. Stretching exercises, yoga, and Pilates consist of gradual movements what can help to active this movement. These exercises are also beneficial because they work every tiny muscle surrounding a joint. Yoga balance postures can help restore the most inhibited joints. It creates a combination of strength and flexibility that significantly reduces pain and improves function/mobility.

Stretching also improves muscular balance and posture by realigning tissue and thereby reducing the effort it takes to maintain good posture throughout the day. Flexible joints require less energy to move through a more excellent range of motion. This decreases your overall risk of injury and increase physical performance as well. Stretching works towards reading resistance in muscle tissue during any activity. Many intense athletes depend on yoga to keep their body from falling apart. I have a marathon friend that could not keep going without it. Again, the yang needs the yin to keep the body in balance.

What if I can't do yoga?

I honestly think there is yoga for everyone. It is far superior to any other stretching techniques. You can do classes at a local studio, generic gyms offer classes, and you can even buy DVD's or watch it on YouTube. The P90X yoga is my favorite video to this day. Unlike most other physical exercises that work only on a physical level, yoga involves both your mental and physical capabilities. There is a balance of energy between the body and the brain while increasing your flexibility, toning your muscles, and improving your lung capacity. Most studios even offer elderly classes that use chairs at props for those unable to do most poses.

If after that, you are still not sold on yoga, please still incorporate stretching into your daily routine. Flexibility exercises should be incorporated into any exercise program. Stretching is best done post-exercise in order to mobilize tight joints from your sport. There are many guided stretching videos available as well. In Crossfit we use ROMWOD.

There are many versions of this available on youtube. Before your workouts it is best to do something called dynamic stretching. This basically means movement stretching. Examples would be arm circles, leg kicks, but kicks, skipping, bear crawls, etc. Do things that warm up the joints, not slow cooling stretches like hamstring stretches. Slow stretches like touching your toes for extended periods can actually increase the risk of injury such as a pulled hamstring when performed before running.

I know this can all get slightly confusing if you are not following a structured program made by a trainer. This is one reason I recommend finding an expert when aiming to improve fitness. Most things in health are done more efficiently when programmed by a professional. I always have patients that are trying to do it all on their own. I was that person. It is a great person to be because at least you are taking responsibility and trying to better the health for you and your family. However, you will get better results with help. When I was self-diagnosing, creating my own exercise programs, and randomly trying diets there were times I did more harm than good. Joining specialized gyms and seeking help from a Functional Medicine doctor helped focus me on diets and exercises that were specific to my own physiology. It helped me cut out all the B.S. that did not apply to me.

Functional Medicine

"Physicians think they are doing something for you by labeling what you have as a disease." -Immanuel Kant

The United States is ranked 37th in healthcare by the WHO (World Health Organization). We have more hospital admissions for preventable disease than comparable countries. We also take more drugs than all other countries combined. Clearly our western medicine approach to healthcare is not working. Our life expectancy is actually decreasing. We need to make some changes in how we view and treat disease. One new approach is called Functional Medicine. Functional medicine is a different philosophy on healthcare.

Functional medicine differs from traditional in the approach towards the body; it looks at a person as a single entity, and it believes that everything is interconnected. Functional medicine attempts to find out the root cause of the ailment, it analyses the triggers that led to the present condition and pays specific attention to the characteristics of the patient so as to provide a personalized remedy. For example, I have many patients with digestive dysfunction. I do not think I have put two people on the same protocol. Some need help with carbohydrate, some with protein. Some have leaky gut, others simply have brain based issues. I could never say, you have gut problems so you get X, Y and Z. Each person is too different in the root cause and their needs.

Getting to Know You

Functional medicine (FM) pays specific attention to the patient's history; it tries to track the origin of the disease. Any chronic condition starts much earlier than it is reported, something that even allopathy has begun to accept. Now, most researchers recognize that diabetes exists at least a decade before being diagnosed, and the same is true for neurodegenerative diseases. Researchers firmly agree that chronic diseases are the result of faulty lifestyle practiced for years or even decades. Many patients will act like their condition just came out of nowhere. That is only because they ignored the red flags the body was trying to wave for them. With the diabetes example, an FM doctor would find pre-diabetes in blood work or recognize symptoms such as headaches in the afternoon, light headed, crashing after meals and insomnia as early signs to address before disease develops.

However, albeit all the progress and understanding, allopathy (traditional medicine) rarely tries to correct the root causes. It looks at the immediate symptoms and alterations in body functions. Thus in diabetes, it gives drugs to control glucose or anti-seizure medications to keep neuropathy in check. Functional medicine is evidence-based medicine with different opinions and outlooks. It sees illness as a reaction or change that occurs due to interaction with the environment. It tries to remove poor environment, thus trying to get rid of the cause and therefore, tries to cure the system.

With the diabetes example again, functional medicine doctors would make nutrition recommendations, evaluate for certain deficiencies, coach on exercise, or see if some other imbalance is causing the diabetes. Each individual is unique, living and interacting with unique micro-environment, having a unique lifestyle and influencing factors. Despite an understanding of the uniqueness of patients, genetics, and environment, allopathy has a "one size fits all" approach. On the other hand, functional medicine understands that lifestyle choices and specificity of interaction with the environment by individuals play a central role in disease development, modification, and alteration of its course. Interaction with the environment may also change the behavior of the gene leading to changes in the body. FM addresses all contributing factors to eliminate disease states.

A word on genetics:

Family history is useful in identifying pathologies to which an individual may be predisposed. HOWEVER, your body is not a machine, it is a complex ecosystem. Ecosystems change and evolve due to environmental stressors, machines do not. Therefore, you control what genes your body expresses based on what internal and external environments you create. Epigenetics has taught us that genes have on and off switches determined by environment that discourages the activation of pathological genetics. Therefore, if you think you are doomed by your genetics, fear not. Environment consists of all the chemical, mental and physical factors we discuss in this book.

Why do doctors not all work this way?

There are many reasons that typical physicians are restricted from practicing similar to functional medicine. One, insurance companies dictate care/cost and coaching takes too much time. Two, pharmaceutical commercials brainwash patients into asking for quick fixes from their doctors so their doc cannot coach properly on lifestyle changes. Therefore, doctors that want to do functional Medicine end up getting out of the insurance world in order to create the time and freedom to treat their patients in this manner.

Functional medicine is not something that is against modern pharmaceutical drugs or allopathic medicine. It tries to compliment it, providing the best of various systems. Thus, functional medicine tries to cure diseases through lifestyle modification, exercise, dietary changes, use of high-quality food supplements, and even pharmacological drugs when required.

Allopathic medicine is excellent at acute care, while functional medicine is about disease prevention, finding the root causes of the diseases, detoxification, metabolism correction, and disease reversal. Thus, if a person had a heart attack, allopathic medicine would help to save a life, but once the condition has stabilized, functional medicine can help to identify the causes of worsening cardiac health, high blood pressure, high cholesterol and help to correct the faulty lifestyle and assist in disease reversal. It can greatly help with the treatment of diabetes, asthma, food allergies, celiac disease, autoimmune diseases, mood disorders, and much more.

Functional medicine is for anyone who wants to get rid of the disease altogether, rather than just continuing to subdue the symptoms.

But what do FM docs do at a visit?

It is always intimidating to meet a new kind of doctor. When seeing an FM doc you do not have to fear that they are going to come at you with crystals, magic wands or dream catchers. Although, I do think my patients expect me to bust out the magic wand sometimes with the supernatural progress they expect to make in one visit. There are six things these doctors will use to diagnose or treat you.

1-Communication-Most information a doctor needs to treat you can be found in a thorough consultation.

2-Blood Work- Normal blood work values are compared to a pool of values collected from usually "sick" individuals. Functional values aim to compare you to "healthy" individuals. We do this by using values that are one or two standard deviations from the average. Normal blood work values encompass over two standard deviations from the mean.

3-Symptom Survey Forms- This is an extensive worksheet of 300 plus symptoms you may encounter in your life. The pattern of these tells the doctor the primary area that needs support.

4-Reflex Points/Muscles- Many areas of the body become tender and dysfunctional with certain organ dysfunction. Have you heard that left arm goes numb during a heart attack? That is not the only mysterious muscle/nerve issue caused by an organ.

5-Lifestyle- You will be instructed on things you can change in your daily routine to heal your body and avoid future symptoms. This can be changes in diet, exercise, relationships, stress, jobs, etc. Basically, this book is covering the things an FM doc will discuss with you.

6-Supplements- These can be used permanently to boost genetic deficiencies. However, most supplements are aimed to support your body until you reach the next level of physical adaptation. Supplements should not be used as a crutch for a poor lifestyle; then they are no different than a pharmaceutical. Changes in lifestyle are paramount to fully fix physiology.

Why do I feel sick if my doctors and/or lab tests say I am normal?

I like to refer to this as having chronic "I don't feel good-itis." It is unnecessary to go through life struggling to enjoy your day due to obnoxious symptoms. Many symptoms may be masked by an Advil, Benadryl, or Pepcid. However, long term use of such substances can be detrimental. With a functional health approach, the root cause of these symptoms will be addressed and studied. For example, instead of using a heartburn medication, digestion may be aided by boosting digestive enzymes or re-aligning the stomach and the brain's communication to it.

But my doctor says I am healthy...

"Healthy" people by today's paradigm can often have significant dysfunction as indicated on a system/symptom survey and functional blood work. These often overlooked "there is nothing wrong, it is all in your head" symptoms may be red flags for undetected illness or pre-disease states. **Not having a diagnosed disease does not mean you are healthy or that you cannot be helped!**

We have so many patients that feel relieved when they get into our office simply because we care to get them back to THEIR normal, not normal defined by medical standards. I have patients break down crying in my office on a daily basis before I even treat them. They cry because I listen and I believe them. I value the information they give and use it to help them get better. I do not just waive off their symptoms as hypochondriac nonsense. I also help the patient understand WHY they are having the symptom in the first place. For example, insufficient protein intake leads to overall muscle weakness. This simple fact is often overlooked by traditional medicine. This person will likely be given some nonsense diagnosis like fibromyalgia, when really they just need to add eggs to their morning routine. I have had patients with this complaint admit to me that they have not eaten protein in 4 days (not even vegan patients). If I did not have protein for a week I would probably be bed-ridden. It is an essential nutrient. If it is missing, there are consequences and usually in muscle seems muscle is made of proteins primarily. It is simple physiology such as this that your FM doctor can help you understand. Of course there are much more complex cases that exist between genetics, multifaceted histories, and injuries but that at least should give you an idea of what FM does for a patient.

Assignments

-Try 30 days of stretching/ yoga

-Make an appointment with a Functional Medicine Doctor.

-Find a meditation technique that fits your lifestyle or at minimum download a quick meditation app to your phone.

Month 8

Leaky Gut, Gut-Brain Barrier, and How Pain Works

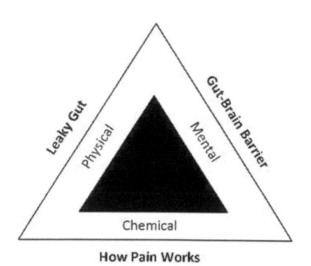

How Pain Works

My Experience

Prior to addressing my gut I am pretty sure I had undiagnosed IBS. I had food reactions that were unpredictable. I had "race to the outhouse" syndrome during exam times and boards. My first Chiropractic Boards I was terrified to take them. I was not scared of the material. I was paranoid that I would need to run to the bathroom. I did not eat breakfast prior to the exam for fear of this phenomenon. You could not leave your seat during these exams. During this test and many other situations, I had every restroom mapped out just in case. If I had to go, I had to go.

Shortly after this low point in my bowel health is when I found Dr. Huff and started a leaky gut program. After the first 30 day program I noticed I did not have to use the bathroom every time I exercised or got stressed. I no longer had bloating. My allergies improved. I did not fall asleep during class. I was more motivated. I had less pain. I even slept better. I had not realized that most of my sleep problems were simply from an upset stomach from gas. The supplement and food program I used and I still use with my patients, was a game changer. I learned how much my gut affected my brain and overall well being.

Even presently I know when my mental health starts to falter that I probably have been pushing my dietary limits too hard. For example, in times when we were rebuilding our office or purchasing other practices, I did the thing where coffee became a meal and lunch was not existent. I ate most of my food past 7PM. I basically did all the things I tell patients not to. When this becomes my habit, my bowels fall apart. I get stomach pain. My skin gets itchy and rashy. My wrists get carpal tunnel. My knee hurts. I start to have wicked emotional swings. I am not sure if I want to cry or punch a wall sometimes. I basically push myself into a leaky gut/brain situation through stress and poor eating habits that come with it.

I feel so blessed that I have to tools to correct this dysfunctional pattern. When I realize my health is regretting the lifestyle decisions I have made I go back to the leaky gut diet and principles discussed here. I can put myself back on track fairly quickly. I always get the question, "Do I have to stay on this diet forever?" and the answer is no. However, if you self-sabotage and put yourself back into a bad gut/brain situation, you may need to revisit this program now and again.

Gut Diseases

There are many symptoms and diagnoses out there surrounding the health of the gut lining. We have Crohn's, Celiac, Irritable Bowel (IBS), Ulcerative Colitis, Diverticulitis, Hemorrhoids, GERD, Fissures, and Exocrine Pancreatic Insufficiency to name a few. So what is the cause of these dysfunctions? That is the discussion that is left out of most doctors' visits and pharmaceutical commercials. Why do so many people have IBS and similar symptoms? The answer usually comes down to one of three things:

1-Leaky Gut

2-SIBO (Small intestine Bacterial Overgrowth)

3-Leaky Brain Barrier

Keep in mind; these are all descriptions of mechanisms, not diagnoses. They tell us the reason behind the diagnosis. Why do you have IBS? Why do you have alternating constipation and diarrhea? Why do you have constant brain fog? Why does your brain just not work like it used to? These are the three reasons. We discussed the importance of digestion to overall health back in chapter 3. I think it's time we got a little more in depth on the subject.

Leaky Gut

Leaky gut is a condition where protein and toxins are able to seep through the tight junctions in the gut lining and into the bloodstream. When foreign particles get into the bloodstream the body creates an immune response to try to protect itself from foreign invaders. This response results in inflammation throughout the body and subsequently creates widespread dysfunction. Leaky gut symptoms include: hormone imbalance, constipation, diarrhea, eczema, joint pain, gut pain, depression, brain fog, malabsorption, and more.

Leaky gut can be caused by a variety of factors including: insufficient enzymes, toxic diet, food intolerances, extreme stress, hormone replacement, over-exercise, gut infections and more.

Treating Leaky Gut involves multiple facets. It comes down to the 4 R's. Remove, replace, repair, replenish. You must remove the poor diet and remove bad bacteria. Replace the diet with healthy and gut friendly foods. The gut lining must be repaired with immune boosting compounds. The gut bacteria must be replenished with probiotics. There are multiple companies with great protocols for this, we use Apex Energetics. For a food list to follow, see the Leaky Gut Food Protocol Located in the Appendix.

SIBO (Small Intestine Bacterial Overgrowth)

Small intestine bacterial overgrowth is another very common gut condition in alternative healthcare today. It commonly presents as intolerance to carbohydrates or yeast infection/overgrowth. Small intestinal bacterial overgrowth (SIBO) is a conditioned caused by excess sugar in combination with bowel bacterial dysregulation. A good way to test if you have this is the potato test: eat white potatoes in excess for a day and see if it reproduces your symptoms such as gas, bloating, constipation or diarrhea. Otherwise there are breath tests that can check for overgrowth, however, these are often not reliable. Your symptoms are more likely to give you a proper diagnosis. While the presentation can be very similar to leaky gut, SIBO (small intestine bacterial overgrowth) symptoms depend on carbohydrate consumption. These carbohydrates are listed in the FODMAPS section, but a great food protocol for this problem moderate to prolonged fasting listed in the appendix. While complete exemption of most carbohydrates is necessary for a successful fix to this problem, other treatments will speed up the process and keep you from reverting. In order to heal SIBO lifestyle, structure, and diet changes must be made.

Common symptoms include:

Abdominal bloating
Constipation
Diarrhea
Acid reflux/GERD Abdominal pain
Weight loss/gain Nutritional deficiencies Leaky Gut
Unexplained swelling
body odor
Bad breath/halitosis belching burping gas Irritable Bowel
Food intolerances
Chronic Pain Depression
Asthma
Allergies
Auto-immune
Fatigue
Mal-absorption
Nausea
Anemia
Fatty stool

Most SIBO is caused by an open Ileo-cecal valve (ICV), discussed in chapter 3. This is a valve between the small and large intestine. It is normal to have high bacteria count in the large intestine, however, when this valve is kept open, many "probiotics" climb to where they do not belong in the small intestine. Therefore, fixing the ICV problem is necessary to healing SIBO. There are many chiropractic protocols that influence the position of the ICV, I recommend seeing an Applied Kinesiology Chiropractor. The ICV also gets stuck open due to gas in the gut. ONE MUST ELIMINATE GAS TO HEAL SIBO! Eliminating gas can help the ICV to open and close as needed. To eliminate gas one must avoid gas producing foods as are listed for SIBO, as well as take as many enzymes as are necessary to eliminate gas formed from allowed foods. There is a full SIBO food protocol list in the appendix.

Another reason for SIBO is a lack of Vagus nerve activity, lack of digestive juices, a decrease in bowel motility, or lack of chill time all leading to undigested food sitting around in the small intestine for too long. There are simple exercises that can increase vagal nerve activity. Gargling water hard while humming Happy Birthday, gagging with a tongue depressor (without vomiting), and chiropractic care are good examples. In order to increase bowel motility, Coffee enemas can be a good exercise. The fullness reflex will help the gastric muscles engage. I would encourage the technique and equipment used in the Gerson Therapy (a lemon water can be used before coffee for best results). See further instructions in appendix. One assignment this month is to choose a Vagus nerve exercise to practice.

There are also many techniques for increasing digestive enzymes. Again, seeing an Applied Kinesiology Chiropractor can help with this problem.

These practitioners can aid in changing a Hiatal Hernia. Hiatal Hernias can compromise digestion due to the uncomfortable position of the stomach against the diaphragm, it is when a section of the stomach is being squeezed by the diaphragm muscle sphincter. Stomach breathing can also decrease the likelihood of a hiatal hernia position of the stomach.

For the short term, digestive enzymes and stomach acid (HCL) can be taken supplementally as well. However, if one wants to avoid a lifetime dependency on these products, there are steps to be taken. Some are: Chewing food more thoroughly, not drinking water with meals, de-stressing around meal time, eating in a relaxed environment, decreasing caffeine dependency, eating less carbs, avoid TUMS and similar products, drink less alcohol, eliminating stomach ulcers and infections, and just eating slower are great ways to optimize digestion.

Stuffy Nose and Sinus Problems

One seemingly unrelated but common symptom of SIBO is a chronically stuffy nose. The lining of the sinuses are just an extension of the gut. The same bacterium affects both. Many chronic sinus issues are due to yeast infection and sugar intake. One addition that can help the sinuses specifically is a neti pot with cirti drops from Micro-balance. 1-2 drops of this essential oil may help clear bad bacteria from the sinus area. SIBO can lead to bacterial overgrowth in the sinuses. Most Netty Pots can be purchased at any pharmacy and come with instructions. I recommend buying the salt to go with it. Another barrier that runs in parallel to the gut lining and sinus lining is the gut-brain barrier.

Gut Brain Barrier

Gut health is important for the absorption of nutrients, that much is obvious. However, the gut has far reaches in the overall function of the body. It plays a vital role in hormone production, thyroid health, and it is extremely interconnected with brain function. The nutrients it absorbs are needed to produce neurotransmitters. In fact, up to 80% of Serotonin is made here. That is your feel good chemical. The gut also plays a vital role in protecting the brain. The gut barrier runs parallel in function to the brain barrier. If one fails the other fails, leading to leaky gut as well as leaky brain.

Gut Brain Communication

There is a two way communication between the gut and the brain. The brain controls the majority of the "rest and digest" system. It influences gut movement, nutrient delivery to organs, body weight, enzyme release and more. The gut sends nutrients to the brain and communicates via nerve pathways and neurotransmitters. Sometimes we must treat the gut, sometimes the brain and neurotransmitters.

Neurotransmitter Symptoms

A decrease in any neurotransmitter can be caused by leaky gut/brain. Neurotransmitters can also be affected by: adrenal fatigue, hypoglycemia, anemia, low mineral status, insufficient protein intake, heavy metal exposure, or insufficient digestive enzymes. Let's discuss some of the most common symptoms and how to increase each "brain hormone" group.

Catecholamines: Low leads to food cravings, addictions, substance abuse, anger, impulsive, high risk behavior. High leads to schizophrenia, aggression, anxiety, high blood pressure, irregular heartbeat, paranoia, chronic pain

Dopamine: Low leads to trouble waking up, low sex drive, restless legs, Parkinson's, cold hands/feet, impulsive, mental/physical fatigue, depressed, apathetic, lack of enthusiasm, ADHD, carbohydrate cravings and lack of concentration.

Serotonin: Low leads to typical depression, constipation, moody, fearful, lack of relaxation feeling, decrease learning ability and focus, lack of well-being sense, insomnia

Melatonin: Serotonin is one chemical reaction from becoming melatonin. This is why serotonin is very needed to control sleep. Low melatonin leads to impaired sleep cycles as well as a lack of regenerative sleep.

GABA: chronic pain, fibromyalgia, cold hands/feet, heart palpitations, tight and stiff feeling, feel overwhelmed, sensitive to light and chemicals, racing thoughts that keep you from sleep, easily agitated, inability to loosen up

Acetylcholine: memory trouble, trouble understanding, lack of passion, forgetful, loses things often, disorientation, dry mouth, constipation, slow thinking, make stupid mistakes

Neurotransmitter Corrections

Consistent rules for correcting brain imbalance is to address leaky gut/brain, balance blood sugar, address anemia, decrease stress, eat adequate protein and fat per body weight, balance hormones and eat more methylated B vitamins. Each neurotransmitter is made from specific amino acids. Amino acids are a component of protein. Here are some more neurotransmitter specific recommendations and the amino acid that goes with each.

- **Catecholamines:** The amino acid tyrosine is high in cheese, edamame, fish, eggs, nuts, seaweed, tofu, and turkey. Stimulants can also increase this one: coffee, cola, tea, chocolate, and spicy food. You must also normalize insulin response to get tyrosine to brain.

- **Dopamine:** The amino acid phenylalanine is high in beef, cheese, chocolate, eggs, fish, oats, pork and turkey.

- **Serotonin:** The amino acid Tryptophan is rich in beef, chicken, fish, turkey, tofu, lamb, liver, spinach, and mushrooms. Serotonin is also dependent on sunlight exposure. That is why we get seasonal depression.

- **Melatonin:** To boost this you must regulate circadian rhythm, boost serotonin, avoid stimulating activity at night, avoid hypoglycemia, and eat protein/fat snack before bed

- **GABA:** Balance progesterone, balance blood sugar, decrease fight or flight, decrease stimulating activities or drugs, evaluate anemia, no oxygen will cause stress, evaluate inflammation, circulation, and oxidative stress, avoid hypoglycemia

- **Acetylcholine:** In order to boost you must increase intake of healthy fats and cholesterol, Acetyl L carnitine, balance glucose, and balance estrogen/testosterone.

NOTE: if you have too many of any neurotransmitter, it is likely due to inflammation. Certain inflammatory cytokines inhibit neurotransmitter breakdown by shutting off the enzymes responsible for ending the signal.

Fat Absorption

The brain is a very fatty organ. It consists of 60% fat. That is why low Fat diets induce depression and memory problems. Especially cholesterol is required for axon health and transmission of signals. Fat keeps the nerves healthy; the most important gut-brain nerve is the vagus.

Vagal Nerve Importance to any gut dysfunction

The Vagus nerve activates the gut and sends blood there. Adequate blood flow is needed to absorb nutrients, create muscle contraction, and to replenish the gut lining. This nerve is also in charge of parasympathetic activity (aka rest and digest). This system can be overridden by fight or flight and that is the reason that stress causes constipation and other gut discomfort. Stress can also increase muscle tension and pain.

How Pain Works

It is important that we first classify pain as an emotion. It's something that is perceived differently by each and every person. You could expose 10 people to the same injury and you would get 10 different responses all requiring separate treatments. Some can bash themselves up really good and just keep on trucking while others would be debilitated from the same injury. Emotion and trauma history plays a huge role in perceived pain. For example, abuse victims almost always perceive pain more severely. Those with depression often feel pain more as well.

Our minds are powerful over our physical symptoms. Oftentimes, there is not even an injury in the area of pain on any measurable test. Unfortunately, when this happens, people's pain goes un-addressed. It is viewed as all in the head. My argument to this is as follows: even if it is a brain based issue, why would you still not try to find the root cause of the problem to try and improve the patient's quality of life? Physical injury or not, there is still a flaw in physiology here that needs to be treated to get the patient back to their normal. Regardless of injury or not, pain changes lives. Relief from it always improves the quality of life.

Pain Pathway

Simply speaking, pain is perceived by nerves and the input travels to the spinal cord, up the spine, and to the brain. However, the chemicals present in the spinal cord and brain dictate how the pain is perceived in intensity. The point of injury decides the quality of the pain. For example, muscles cause dull and achy pain. Nerve can be described as shooting, burning or tingling. Lack of communication with the brain is described as weakness more than pain. There is variability in the circuits in different individuals that determine the pain experience.

Sometimes pain even switches sides. This is due to a spillover of chemicals in the spinal cord which can lead the brain to perceive pain on the wrong side. There are many instances with rotator cuff tear patients where the tear seen on an MRI is on the opposite side of the pain. Of course, this may also be due to compensating for the weak/torn side. We more often experience pain from overuse than an underused/injured one.

We also tend to have a lot of ignored/hidden pain or injuries. The brain is really great at promoting survival. Often enough, this requires ignoring discomfort. The Salient network of the brain dictates what to pay attention to. This is for obvious reasons. If we are trying to escape a predator, who cares if the knee hurts? You got to keep running. I have a number of patients that have been in fight or flight so long from chronic pain that they are unaware of multitudes of dysfunction. We will get their back pain under control and all of a sudden that have neck pain. This is not a weird phenomenon. The neck dysfunction had always been there. The back was simply to greater priority to the Salient system. Once the back was healed, the next area of dysfunction could be concentrated on.

Food and Pain

Nutritional status has everything to do with perceived pain. We have discussed how inflammation causes pain. I always get confused remarks from patients such as "I had really bad pain Wednesday, Thursday and Friday I thought it was gone, then Saturday was unbearable" or "doc, I just do not understand why some days are so much worse." The answer is inflammation and/or nutritional deficiencies. I have seen a number of "fibromyalgia" patients that were really just depleted of Omega 3 and cholesterol from too long of low-fat dieting. If your pain is due to inflammation, it should have been thoroughly addressed by all preceding chapters.

There are times pain is literally just muscle fatigue from inadequate nutrients. This will be discussed more in chapter 15 but let's look at one scenario. If you go to the gym and hit a personal record on your squat and do not have ample protein that day, you will barely be able to get up off the toilet the next day and you will hurt all over. I see this happen over and over in my office (just minus the squat PR). People will have extremely active days and barely eat protein. Whether you are a weight lifter or not, your muscles still need protein for recovery. So if you have a muscle injury and are only eating pasta and bread every day, do not expect to recover in any reasonable time. If I asked you, "when is the last time you ate protein," and you couldn't answer or ask if a 200 calorie protein bar counts then you will feel like trash. Therefore, if you are in pain after a long day at your physical job, you may just need to eat a steak to get out of pain.

Emotions and Pain

Your emotional stress plays a huge part in this as well. For example, loneliness causes increased pain perception. This is one of many reasons we feel pain when we lose a loved one. On a less depressing note, freshman in college will experience a lot more health issues after leaving home. Junk food and booze are not the only culprits. Loneliness is a huge factor.

On the flip side of emotions causing pain, pain can change emotions and even personality. The brain and spinal cord change with chronic pain patients. There is a spill-over of a lot of chemicals from pain that can affect the frontal lobe which controls our behavior. Pain is also exhausting. It completely burns out the nervous system. My coworker in one office had words that really stuck with me. "Never judge a patient on day one in the office. Their brain does not work. The pain can make them obstinate and slightly mad." Never judge another's pain level. You do not walk in their shoes and have no idea what they are experiencing.

Pain affects everyone differently. Some people are affected more than others. To some it is a distraction. They cannot get through their day or perform any normal activities. Some people power through it and use it as a motivator to finish a task faster, or use tasks to distract them from pain. We all cope in our own way. With coping you let go endorphins, called runners high in some cases. If you are not coping, find a way to. Many get a runners high from chiropractic care for this reason.

Some people may need cognitive behavioral techniques to release these issues. This may require professional counseling. Remember, the mental component of the triangle of health is very important. You may think you pain is all physical and that is far from the truth. EVERYONE has an emotional component to their pain.

Pain Treatment Efficacy

The best pain relief is the one you believe in. This is a great rule to live by with any medical treatment. Whether you think ibuprofen, peppermint oil, CBD oil, Mary Jane, laser, acupuncture, chiropractic, massage, or steroids help your pain, you are probably right. Even if the pain relief technique you prefer is highly un-researched or just plain crazy, it still works. There are no if, ands, or buts about it. I will tell you why. The placebo effect can actually have measurable therapeutic outcomes. Placebo works 18%-80% of the time. Rogaine studies had men regrow hair that were just getting sugar pills. On the flip side of that, you must be weary of believing what you hear about any treatment being negative too. Nocebo is when patients feel side effects without getting the true treatment. Cancer patients given saline solution instead of chemo actually threw up and started losing hair because they believed it would happen if they were actually getting chemo.

Moral of this story: The power of suggestion is very strong. It can produce positive or negative health benefits. Therefore, you should be sure you have a belief in the treatment you are pursuing or it will not work regardless of how many research studies were performed with it. In order to get rid of any pain condition, one needs to eliminate the negatively biased mind and start to believe in the possibility of recovery.

Stress and Pain

Chronic tension leads to chronic pain. Stress increases pain because adrenaline increased muscle tension. You have likely experienced some degree of this in your life. When we experience stress of anxiety, we all tend to clench jaws and shrug up our shoulders. When this is done for days or months on end, it leads to neck pain and headaches. Now while some of us go through this a few times a year, chronic/ongoing pain can happen when a person gets stuck in this cycle. Certain traumas can allow us to fall into this chronic tension state. Or there is the most obvious, chronic stress that can produce this problem.

The complete elimination of this kind of pain may require a change in lifestyle. Depending on the stressor, professional help may be required to fully address. We can do a method called Emotional Balance Technique in our office that incorporates positive affirmations with acupressure points. However, I still suggest seeing a counselor.

Assignments

Follow a gut repair diet for the month.

Engage in Vagal Nerve exercise

Identify an emotional stressor that affects your wellness or pain levels and seek professional help

Month 9

Massage, Household Chemicals, and Putting Yourself First

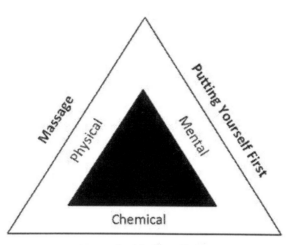

Household Chemicals

My Experience

So my husband and I have on ongoing joke about how much I sneeze in the morning. He counts and makes bets on how many I will get. I recently noticed, I do not sneeze when I do not wear perfume, hair spray, or other strong odor products. I used to think it was just because my body needed to clear some stuff out first thing in the morning. I have since tested this theory. Every time I treat a patient that wears too much cologne, I sneeze. Weird factory odor, I sneeze.

Now I would love to call this an allergy but sneezing is the only symptom. I am pretty convinced it is just my body rejecting toxic chemical exposure. There are a number of weird and questionable ingredients in many "hygiene" products. I now have ditched the perfume, started buying alternative deodorants, make-up, shampoo, house cleaners, etc.

Household Chemicals

It is important to monitor your chemical exposure for many reasons. Obviously we have a whole chapter on detoxification. There is less need to detoxify if you have a low amount of exposure to gunk in the first place. While work exposure and our outdoor world are difficult to control, we can control what is on our own home. The most abundant, possibly contaminated, compound in your house is the water. You drink it, clean with it, bathe in it; it's a constant bombardment.

Water Quality

We are swimming in a sea of estrogen. From agriculture to birth control, estrogen is everywhere. Estrogen excess can cause cancer, make men more feminine, interrupt normal female menstrual cycle, lead to excess menstrual bleeding and cramping, cyst formation, PCOS, leaky gut, various types of cancer (breast, ovarian, colorectal, prostate, endometrial), osteoporosis, neurodegenerative diseases, cardiovascular disease, insulin resistance, lupus erythematosus, endometriosis, and obesity. One of the reasons water quality is important is to be sure you are not getting excess hormones. There are many additional reasons to get a water purification system. A few toxin examples are lead, chlorine, fluoride, pesticides, insecticides, fuel additives, and industrial chemicals. I know water in my town has so much chlorine it tastes like pool water. Actually, it pretty much is pool water. My dad tested the tap water with the chlorine reader for the hot tub and it verified we were drinking pool water levels of chlorine.

We buy Culligan water in our town. There are many great systems out there. We just love the convenience of the water cooler in our waiting room and kitchen. I love having cold water without the trouble of using ice. I also think this water tasted better than the tainted tap water. It even makes the coffee taste better. Most popular coffee places will filter their water because they know that it affects taste.

I constantly have patients that do "not like water." I think this goes against physiology and don't really understand. You can go a month without food and survive or more. You can only make it days without water or you die. Water is vital. However, if the taste just doesn't fit your fancy, spice it up a bit. You can use a drop of peppermint oil, squeeze a lemon, soak a cucumber in it, or just add any fruit. There are also many herbal teas that taste great. We like to make "sun tea" in the summer. Just add a few bags of your favorite flavor to a pitcher of water and sit in the sun for a few hours.

Ways to Control Our Water

The typical sink and pitcher filters will remove some chlorine but not hormones and heavy metals. We use a reverse osmosis system in our house and office. It takes out the chlorine best as well as drugs and agriculture chemicals. You can also choose from alkaline water systems or deionization filters. They all have their own benefits. Deionized water removes everything. This can be helpful for certain cleanses and heavy metal detox.

What is alkaline water? Water is supposed to be neutral, around a PH of 7. However, there are many water brands out there or tap waters out there that can be dangerously acidic. I do not want to shout out brand names here but watch the YouTube video "Is you water acidic or alkaline?" Buying or creating the proper PH of water is helpful. Alkaline water systems will take it a step further and get your water to about 9.5 PH. The benefit in this is that the stressful, poor diet, and pollution laden lives we live can be very acidic and somewhat balanced out by our water if we buy alkaline.

The Lie of Bottled Water

Don't go rushing for bottled water. Many companies just use tap water and sell it bottled. Not to mention the un-excusable amount of waste produced from bottles and other plastics and the fact that the plastics leach into the bottled water. If you are purchasing the refillable water jugs, shoot for spring water. Distilled has literally everything removed and will not quench your thirst. You do want some electrolytes kept in your water. Electrolytes are magnesium, sodium, calcium, phosphorus, etc.

Plastic Waste

We need to take better care of our planet regardless of which side of the global warming argument you fall on. We need to support the companies that are creating less waste and less toxic chemicals so that we have a beautiful place to live for a while longer. I think the best way to do so is in reducing plastic waste. Anytime you can you should bring reusable grocery bags. Bring your own coffee mug. Use glass Tupperware instead of plastic bags for your food. You do not have to be a recycling Nazi to do your part. Plastic bags are what I concentrate on most. Anytime they give me a to-go bag for one burrito bowl. I about lose my mind. I can carry my one bowl without the giant bag that could fit 5 meals. I always get the weirdest look when I deny that bag. We need to start changing that. Our food system is where we all create the most volume of waste.

So bring your own containers/bags whenever possible. For example, stop double bagging your damn vegetables. I know I tick off the check-out counter because I bring my avocados up naked and I do not care. Really though, you usually use an extra 5-10 plastic bags for no reason just in the fruit/veggie isle.

Essential Oils

Another way to reduce waste and toxins is to change your cleaning products. There is a lot of scrutiny over the efficacy of essential oils and natural products for medicinal purposes. I do not care where you stand on that topic, there is no arguing that household chemicals are dangerous and essential oils provide obvious benefit as an alternative. You can make your own cleaning solution with a simple base of vinegar and water and any oil for scent. Certain citrus oils are particularly good at removing sticky icky stuff. Any such concoction is safe for anyone in your home. We all forget about vinegar and other household basics. Prior to popular cleaning brands hitting the shelf, vinegar and baking soda were to cleaning essentials. Baking soda is great for many things. My favorite is for soaking up spills or accidents from the carpet. Baking soda can soak up moisture and odors.

The most obvious reason to switch to an alternative cleaner is child/pet safety. You do not have to rush to the hospital if your child drinks vinegar with lavender oil in it. You would be rushing to the ER if they got into the bleach or toilet scrubbers. The second reason to go natural is to reduce your toxic load/exposure.

Even if you do not create your own essential oil concoctions, there are many premade available at health food stores. Even the basic cleaners at the grocery store labeled environmentally friendly are better than the generic toxin loaded ones.

Oils should be used for diffusing as well instead of the typical plug ins. Oils can be used just for ambiance. They are much cleaner than the estrogenic scents used in most air fresheners. The same goes for perfume scents too. Most body sprays are extremely toxic and can negatively affect your brain.

Top 5 Oils for Cleaning

Thieves- This is the ultimate in killing off crud. Use it to kill the bad bugs during cold and flu season.

Orange- Many citrus oils are like goo-gone. They help remove gunk.

Lemon- This gives your house the fresh typical clean smell. It is also great to cut through grease.

Lavender- It is calming and great for laundry scent.

Tea Tree/ Melaleuca- This is very antiviral, antifungal, and anti-bacterial. It can be used to disinfect your house or for hygiene products.

Hygiene Products

Our skin absorbs what we touch in less than 30 seconds. This sounds crazy but how else would your body know to pull away from a dangerous chemical. Therefore we absorb everything from our shampoo all the way to our laundry detergent.

Personal care products such as deodorant contain aluminum, parabens, and fragrance that mimic estrogen in the body. While many cancers are driven by estrogen, primarily breast cancer, we need to reduce out estrogen-ish compound exposure. Other ingredients to look out for are formaldehyde, SLS (Sodium lauryl sulfate), perfume, BHT, PEG compounds, Siloxanes, petrolatum, glycols, Dibutyl phthalate, and coal tar dyes (CI). You should be conscious of these in your toothpaste, shampoo, deodorant, make-up, nail polish, detergent, fabric softener, soaps, and lotions.

Lotions often contain the most toxic ingredients. I highly recommend using coconut oil for most of your moisture needs. If that doesn't do the trick, animal fat will. My favorite dry skin product in the office has lard as the first ingredient. Generally even your massage therapist will use coconut oil for treatments because they do not want repeated chemical exposure to nasty lotions either.

Massage

One of the major misconceptions about massage is that it is only a relaxation rub down. This is like saying you only go to Starbucks for black coffee. While massage is great for stimulating the parasympathetic rest and digest system, it offers much more than that. Massage treats primarily three systems. It treats muscles, lymph, and nerve. Muscles alone can be injured in multiple mechanical ways that all require different treatment. Lymph contains most of our detoxification processes and immune system cells. Of course the nervous system controls the whole body as discussed in the chiropractic chapter. You may see some parallels with how massage works and how chiropractic works. That is why these two techniques work so well in conjunction. They both target the musculoskeletal system. Chiropractors move the skeletal component while massage concentrates on the muscular. Both techniques have far reaching healing capabilities throughout the body systems.

Much like with Chiropractic, you can address your massage therapist with specific complaints. For example, I have mine help me with my stomach. When I get really stressed, I get a hiatal hernia (my stomach rides upward and gives me heartburn and pain). I tell my therapist of this and she will do a diaphragm release for me to help my digestion. You could also see a masseuse for specific joint pain. If you injure your shoulder throwing a ball, your therapist may spend a half hour alone treating your shoulder injury. As much as it pains me to admit that Chiropractic may not be able to fix any and all things, some people are just better suited for massage. So just because you cannot get adjusted does not mean you need to surrender to pills and shots. Give massage a try. We will be discussing other types of alternative treatments in chapter 14.

Speaking of stress, massage is the most suited profession to address stress induced pain. If you notice that times of high stress cause back pain, headaches, dizziness, heartburn, TMJ, etc., then you really need a massage. I mean this medically. Everyone halfheartedly states that if you are stressed you should get a massage. Even if your friends tell you this as a mild suggestion, take it. Massage is not just a "treat yourself" kind of luxury. There are times it is just plain medically necessary.

Even the Mayo clinic has become a proponent of massage as a medical therapy. While it is known to help muscle tension, stress, and pain, massage also has confirmed benefits for:

- Anxiety

- Digestive Disorders

- Fibromyalgia

- Headaches

- Insomnia

- Sinus Pressure

- Sports Injuries

- Muscle Strains

- TMJ (Temporomandibular Joint Pain)

There are innumerable practices out there for body work. Here are some descriptions of the most common massage techniques:

Swedish Massage- This is a typical relaxation massage technique. It uses gentle kneading, tapping, and circular movements to calm down the tissues. It is aimed to release tension and decrease inflammation.

Trigger Point Massage- Trigger points are usually caused by a decrease in oxygen to a muscle. This technique aims to unwind the tight muscle fibers that are depleting the tissue. This is great for injured or overused muscles. It also helps treat referred pain. For example, tight shoulder muscles can result in neck pain. I have had experiences with massage where I get my glute released and it gets rid of my heartburn. You never know how far reaching these reflexes can be.

Deep Tissue Massage- This type uses slow and high pressure strokes to get into the deep layers of connective tissue. This is great for certain muscle injuries. However, this type tends to really release a lot of inflammatory chemicals that have been stored deep in the tissues. It detoxifies the body. Therefore, you will likely feel some soreness and grogginess after this style. That is why therapists encourage you to drink water afterwards. Certain individuals should be hesitant to get this technique as they may feel worse instead of better. Deeper is not always best. I am talking to you athletes here. It does not have to hurt to benefit you. In fact, most athletes would benefit from less deep tissue as your muscles are abused enough already.

Sports Massage-This is a specific treatment to be used before/after sporting events to prevent injury. It aims to increase range of motion. Depending on if you are pre/post workout the therapist may aim to engage or relax involved muscles.

Thai Massage- This is generally used in Yoga studios as a form of stretching massage. It is aimed to help with joint flexibility.

Hot Stone- This is not what it looks like in spa commercials. You are not just lying around with rocks on your back. Hot stone is actually when the therapist uses the heated stones as a hand tool to get deeper into the muscles. The heat also restores blood flow to help release trigger points and other difficult areas.

One assignment this month is to get a massage each week with a different masseuse. Much like with chiropractors, each masseuse is different. There are different techniques, styles and skills involved. Figure out what works for you. Do you like deep pressure? Hot stone? Swedish? Thai? Sports? There are many to try. They all offer different benefits. Always remember, it does not have to be painful to be beneficial. Communicate with your therapist on your preferred pressure, they cannot read your mind.

Putting yourself first

Scheduling a massage each month is an example of putting yourself, and your health, first. A common misunderstanding is that putting yourself first is selfish and self-centered. I challenge you this: if you do not take care of yourself, who will?

Usually those hating on you are doing so because they are jealous. The reason a person does not like another is usually because they see an aspect of themselves in that person that they hate about themselves or they just plain envy what the other has mastered. As an example, I will use my aunt. She had three young boys. She has always spent ample time at the gym. She knows she has to do this to manage her pain and auto-immune disease. She has many times been ridiculed for taking too much time to herself. Other women would call her selfish because they thought she should not be at the gym but instead hanging out with her kids. There are so many flaws in this logic but I will explain a few. One reason the other moms hated on her is because she has a rocking hot body and they are jealous. She also has a fit family, loving children, and an awesome supportive attractive spouse. They are successful and are what I identify as a power family. The women hating on her for her gym time were tearing her down because they all wished they had what she possesses. This is a common thing in society. We hate those who have it better than us. Really what we would do if we were smart is study those we hate or hold jealousy towards. Study their habits so that we could become more like them.

The other flaw in these women hating on her is in the principle that keeping yourself healthy allows you to help others. It is imperative, especially for moms, to put time and effort into your health so that you may take care of your family. If you are not healthy and you are in and out of the hospital and doctor's appointments or are too exhausted to leave your room, you cannot help anyone. So take time for the massage, buy yourself a gym membership, go to the chiropractor, take a day off, etc. I see it often where moms will bring their kids to me before themselves. Usually, their health is far worse than their child's. Not to mention, children absorb their parents' problems. You can see this in anything from back pain, to gut discomfort, to mental illness. Therefore, if the parent does not heal, neither will the child. Now you may think this is all voodoo nonsense but hear me out. When my patient was having marital problems she was very constipated. Her daughter was 2 but apparently keen enough to pick up on the parents' turmoil. She also became very constipated. When the marital problems were addressed they both could poop again. I could have adjusted the child a zillion times and given her every supplement but until the marital problems of the parents were addressed she would not have recovered.

Therefore, parents need to start putting themselves first and it will actually help the children they love most. This can be applied to most caregiver relationships. It is important to put yourself first so that you may better serve others. I recently had a patient that lost a parent. Instead of canceling her appointments, she came in weekly. She remarked to me how happy she was that she had committed to doing something for herself because it helped her through the tough times. She pushed past the guilt of leaving her responsibilities for that few minutes of self-care each week and it kept her going.

One assignment this week is to take a "me day." Take a day and schedule some self-care. This may be getting out of town, shopping, sleeping, massage, nails, overdue doctor's appointments, reading, hunting, hiking, shooting, boating, beaching, or whatever floats your boat.

Assignments

Take a "Me Day"

Schedule a Massage

Detox your cleaning cabinets

Month 10

Ketogenic Diet, Weight Loss, and Mindset

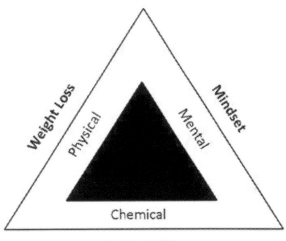

Ketogenic Diet

My Experience

Weight loss for me requires intense focus, tracking everything, and a lot of cardio. I can maintain my weight by following most of the programs in this book and stay healthy. However, if I want to slim down, I have to get my mind right.

The two consistent rules I have found for weight loss personally are 0g of sugar and getting my steps in. In this chapter we will discuss the ketogenic diet which is one type of 0g of sugar approach to weight loss and overall well being. This diet did also help me tremendously with mental health and focus.

Now, just because I know how to lose weight does not mean I do not have times where I get a little sloppy and gain a few. Maintaining weight loss requires the right mindset and avoiding self-sabotage. It also requires constant motivation and self-checks on diet and exercise. There are multiple times a year that I have to put my fitbit on and make sure I am still moving as much as I should. I will also count sugar often to be sure I am not going too far in the wrong direction.

In a society full of the wrong options and multitudes of temptation, there is a lot of mental toughness required to keep a healthy weight. I want to share with you some techniques that have helped me.

Mindset

First of all, if you skipped the whole book to read the weight loss chapter, STOP. Turn around. Go back to the beginning. Most month's programs are designed to heal the body by decreasing inflammation, which will lead to weight loss in most individuals. This chapter is going to be focused more on the calorie intake vs. burn stereotypical weight loss mumbo jumbo. However, many people cannot lose weight without address underlying gut and hormone imbalances discussed earlier on. Moral of the story, follow the book in order and you will be more likely to see transformative results. Also as mentioned earlier, weight driven goals almost always fail. You need to make your health more worthy than what the scale says.

Do not solely concentrate on weight loss, but instead on bettering your overall health. Often enough, when you focus on fixing digestive or other health disturbances you will lose weight in the process. I have had many patients gain muscle and lose fat without a specific exercise or "diet" program. They simply followed one of the previous protocols to fix their diagnosed dysfunction and found good weight loss results in the process. The foods on any/all of these protocols have weight loss potential.

How long should weight loss take?

Most goals in life require more than a 30 day plan. If you have a financial goal, it takes years. If you have a family goal, it takes years. Fitness and sports goals also take years. For some reason we think weight loss should be different. Think about this: my goal is to back squat 300 pounds. This has been a goal of mine for years. I am currently up to 285. I started below 100 years ago. It will probably take me another 6 months to 2 years to hit 300. That is because gaining muscle is an intricate process that takes fuel, time and grit. Weight loss is the same. You cannot expect to squat 300 lbs. in less than a year just like you cannot expect to lose 150lbs. in one year. Weight loss takes time and focused effort. We need to change our mindset.

I always have patients say they only lost 15 lbs. in a month and they are disappointed! They expected to lose more. STOP THIS MENTALITY! Steady sustainable weight loss is only 2-5 lbs. a month for most individuals. Go pick up a 15 lbs. weight. That is the starting weight for most barbells at my gym. That is a substantial amount of weight. If you were to go for a hike with a 15 if backpack vs. without one, you would feel a gargantuan difference. We need to look at weight loss just like that 300 if squat goal. A few pounds a month gradually gets us to our goal. 50-pound jumps in one month are close to impossible. The circumstances that would allow that much weight loss that quick are usually detrimental to your health.

Weight loss requires forced adaptation just like muscle gain requires lifting weights. Lifting weights forces the body to build muscle to be able to better adapt to the load it has been put under. If you want to be lighter, you have to put your body in an environment which makes it think that would be advantageous. For example, running is very dependable with weight loss because your body knows that it would be more metabolically efficient to run at a lighter weight. It's less stress on the joints as well as requiring less calories. You see, weight loss is not always calories in calories out. Usually it's about adaptation. Even with the calorie reduction argument, the reason your body loses weight is because your body's metabolism cannot continue supporting the higher body weight without more calories. Weight loss should always be considered from this standpoint. What can you do to force adaptation?

What Determines Weight Loss

It is when you eat, what you eat, and portion sizes that will determine weight loss. The previous protocols cover the what. You should now know which foods agree with your body. What we have left to discuss is portions and when to eat them. I find generally, that eating more food earlier in the day and less late in the day is more beneficial for physiology as well as weight loss. You burn more calories when the sun is out because our metabolism is greatly dependent on light. That is why our metabolism is slower in winter and we tend to gain weight.

Portion sizes are where things get tricky. Depending on your goals this may require strict regulation. If you want six pack abs, you may need to measure you food with a scale and get exact portions of fat, carbohydrate, and protein. Your exercise regime will also play a part in this. If your goal is in this realm, I recommend finding a nutrition coach to work with you on exact meal plans for your body and exercise type. However, if your goal is simply to fit into your old jeans again and get healthy, portions are easier to manage. Generally, I talk in portion sizes in percentage of your plate. Half of your plate should be vegetables (green, leafy, or non-starchy), a quarter can be starchy veggies, and a quarter will be your protein. Never forget, lots of water throughout the day! Fruit can be used as a snack between meals, but stick to one orange or 1 cup of berries (size of a handful or two). Many will have to completely cut out fruit to lose weight depending on your blood sugar. Exact portions will be discussed more in chapter 15.

Antagonists for Weight Loss

Inflammation, infection, allergies, autoimmune, hormone instability, blood sugar instability, adrenal fatigue, impaired detox, neurotransmitter imbalance, and overtraining can be reasons for weight loss resistance. The most common is insulin resistance. This was thoroughly discussed in the blood sugar chapter. As you will notice, most of these mechanisms have been discussed at length in prior chapters. The second most prevalent reason for weight loss resistance is lack of sleep. Many need 8 hours a night in order to lose weight. There are a few mental blocks for weight loss as well. There are three primary mental challenges:

1-Cheating is OK mentality

Many start a new program and add a cheat meal to try and keep them sane. There are a few flaws in this logic. I know I always stress the 80/20 rule, however, this doesn't mean going completely bonkers with junk. For weight loss, usually 100% effort is required for a month at minimum to see results. If you always think you deserve a "bad" food, it will be hard to give them up. For many personalities, a full elimination is needed in order to quit craving certain foods.

2-Becoming fat adapted

Your body starts to burn your own body fat for fuel once the sugar stores in your tissues are depleted. This is why you learn that fat burning doesn't start until about a half hour of cardio in exercise physiology class. Now, if you are eating a high carbohydrate cheat meal each week, you will replenish your sugar stores and there is no reason for your body to burn body fat for fuel. Sugar is much easier to use. It takes mental grit to say no to sugar and allow adaptation to occur.

3-Leptin Levels

Leptin is what tells your brain that it is full. If you are used to eating large meals to get full, your body requires more leptin to be satisfied. If you want to lose weight, your body needs to adapt to requiring less Leptin. Eating cheat meals will interfere with this connection. If you want to stimulate Leptin without eating mass quantities, eat fat. Fat directly stimulates leptin release. The further you reduce calories and portions, the more toughness it will take to power through the leptin withdrawal.

Understanding water weight

Inconsistent water weight can be a major frustration in weight loss. Water does have weight, therefore if you drink a 16oz bottle of water you will gain a pound temporarily. If you drink 8 cups of coffee, you will gain a few pounds temporarily. That is just the laws of physics. This is one of many reasons I recommend measuring body composition instead of weight alone. If you are using a stereotypical scale (measures weight only), you should weigh yourself first thing in the morning, after using the restroom, before consuming food or water to deter water-weight discrepancies.

Many people will increase muscle mass or water weight during a health program. Building muscle makes you retain water in order to recover from workouts. This initially will make it look like you gained weight but the body composition machines will say you did lose fat. That is important to know. Most overweight/obese individuals are extremely under-muscled. Muscle strength is one of the biggest factors in living to an old age independently. Gaining muscle is always good even if your number on the scale looks larger.

Healthy Composition looks like this:

Body Fat Percentage Chart

	Underfat	Ideal	Overfat	Obese
Woman				
Age 20-39	<21%	<21% to 33%	34% to 39%	>39%
Age 40-59	<23%	<23% to 34%	35% to 40%	>40%
Age 60-79	<24%	<24% to35%	36% to 42%	>42%
Men				
Age 20-39	<8%	8% to 19%	20% to 25%	>25%
Age 40-59	<11%	11% to 21%	22% to 28%	>28%
Age 60-79	<13%	13% to 34%	25% to 30%	>30%

Muscle Mass Percentage Chart

Gender	Age	Low (-)	Normal (0)	High (+)	Very High
	18-40	<24.4	24.4-30.2	30.3-35.2	>35.3
Female	41-60	<24.2	24.2-30.3	30.4-35.3	>35.4
	61-80	<24.0	24.0-29.8	29.9-34.8	>34.9
	18-40	<33.4	33.4-39.4	39.5-44.1	>44.2
Male	41-60	<33.2	33.2-39.2	39.3-43.9	>44.0
	61-80	<33.0	33.0-38.7	38.8-43.4	>43.5

Bone Mass Ranges Chart

Gender	Weight		
Female	Less than 110 lb (50 kg)	110 lb-165 lb (50 kg-75 kg)	165 lb abd up (75 kg and up)
	4.3 lb (1.95 kg)	5.3 lb (2.40 kg)	6.5 lb (2.95 kg)
Male	Less than 143 lb (65 kg)	143 lb -209 lb (65 kg- 95 kg)	209 lb and up (95 kg and up)
	5.9 lb (2.66 kg)	7.3 lb (3.29 kg)	8.1 lb (3.69 kg)

Body Water Chart

Gender	BF% Range	Optimal BW % Range
Male	4-14 %	70-63%
	15-21%	63-57%
	22-24%	57-55%
	25 and over	55-37%
Female	4-20%	70-58%
	21-29%	58-52%
	30-32%	52-49%
	33 and over	49-37%

You must consider each of these factors when evaluating your health. Weight alone tells us very little. For example, most athletes would rate as borderline obese if you looked at their height/weight/BMI alone. With body composition, they may actually be underweight for their size. It can be this drastic due to variances in muscle/water mass.

How to Measure Weight Loss without the Scale

I would like everyone to choose a measurement for their health, besides weight, to use as a goal/indicator. Here are some examples: better mental function, sleep quality, fitting into an old outfit, body fat percentage, seeing muscle definition in a photo, better digestive function, less depression, losing a dress size, etc. This should be charted in your journal. I would also like to stress the photo example, because it is great to have a visual to compare each month. Many will see huge differences in how they look in a bathing suit long before the scale changes since muscle weighs more than fat, yet takes up less space. This is important to track, the more success you feel the more likely you are to stick to a program.

When it comes to measuring weight loss, I find it is best to look at a dexa scan if available or use tape measurements to determine progress rather than just the number on the scale. Getting healthier is more important than weight loss (in pounds). Muscle weighs more than fat so many find that they will shrink into old clothes or see muscle definition before they lose a pound. Shrinking and more muscle mass is the goal, not the number on the scale, especially in those without much to lose.

Ketogenic Diet

Losing weight or attempting to keep fit can feel like a full time job. The market is flooded with a barrage of unhealthy food choices that can easily derail a healthy diet. It is difficult to get enough physical activities to cross-check the calories we consume, that is why hi-jacking our metabolism with a dynamic diet is the best way to reach your fitness potential. Ketogenic Dieting is one of the best ways of dieting for weight loss, brain function, and more.

What is Keto/ketogenic?

It is a diet approach designed to teach your body to use fat for fuel instead of carbohydrates. Hence, you can burn your own body fat for energy. On a typical carbohydrate diet, the body will utilize glucose as the principal source of energy because it is easier to burn. By bringing down the consumption of carbohydrates, the body is actuated into a state known as ketosis. The goal is to hit approximately 70% fat, 20% protein, and 10% carbohydrates. This is unlike the Standard American Diet (SAD diet) which is 40% carbohydrate or more. See appendix for list of fats, proteins, and carbohydrates.

Ketosis is a process the body starts naturally to enable us to survive when consumption of food into the body is low. Amid this state, we create ketones, which are delivered from the breakdown of fats in the liver. The ultimate objective of a carefully kept up ketogenic diet is to drive your body into this metabolic state. We don't do this through starvation of calories only starvation of sugars. Our bodies are extraordinarily versatile to what you put into it – when you overburden it with fats and take away sugars, it will start to consume ketones as the essential vitality source. Ideal ketone levels offer you wellbeing of the body, weight reduction, better physical and mental performance.

The body's metabolism works similar to a fire. A fire burns fuel to create heat and so does our metabolism. Think about this as an analogy; the fat is the logs, the protein is the kindling, and the carbohydrates are the paper. When you put paper on a fire, it burns within a few seconds. Logs however take a while to get going but then burn all night. This is similar to fat metabolism; it takes longer to get going but once the mechanisms are in place your metabolism burns much hotter, longer, and more efficiently. That is the point of reaching ketosis, to burn fat efficiently.

History of the Keto Diet

Ketogenic diet became well known as a treatment for epilepsy in the 1920s. Be that as it may, the diet was long forgotten because of the development of new anticonvulsant drugs. The first logical examination into fasting as a cure for epilepsy was carried out in France, in 1911. The ketogenic diet was found to enhance the patient's psychological capacities.

Fast forward to recent years, some research reveals that a ketogenic diet can be useful to prevent certain infections, Alzheimer's, cancer, epilepsy, and so on. The reason for a few of these is that diseases feed off of sugar. Things like cancer cells can have four times the sugar receptors as regular cells, but most cancer does not metabolize fat for fuel. Also, the brain is a very fatty organ, at 60% fat composition. By fortifying the brain, we may be able to elude certain brain-based diseases.

Since these breakthroughs, our western medicine world has been largely dictated by the pharmaceutical explosion. We are now entering a time where diet changes are paramount to our survival. The millenials are the first generation not expected to outlive their grandparents. Our obsession with drugs must stop, and we must take responsibility and control of what goes into our mouths. It is best we continue this logical search for an optimal diet that can cure our western diseases. With today's knowledge, keto is the most logical way to go for many conditions or genetic predispositions.

What can this help?

Ketogenic diet brings typical glucose levels down due to the kind of food you are expected to consume. Some research demonstrates that the ketogenic diet is a more viable approach to control diabetes, unlike low-calorie diets. In case you're pre-diabetic or have Type II diabetes, you ought to truly consider a ketogenic diet.

Keto also has therapeutic implications with conditions such as:

- Leaky gut
- Small intestine bacterial overgrowth (SIBO)
- Yeast overgrowth
- PCOS
- Infertility
- Arthritis
- Depression / anxiety
- Memory diseases
- Seizures
- Diabetes

How It Works-Monitoring Carb Reduction

Just like many other Low Carb Diets, Ketogenic diets work with the reduction of consumption of glucose. Since most people live on a high carb diet, our bodies ordinarily keep running on glucose (or sugar) for vitality. When glucose is reduced from food consumption, we start to consume stored fat or fat from the food we eat. This mechanism will lead to weight loss.

Since sugar reduction is how it works, sugar must be closely monitored. I recommend using a phone app to track your food at the beginning just to verify where the carbohydrate or glucose molecules are hidden. Some are hidden where you least expect. If you do not monitor your sugar or carbohydrates at the beginning, you may get frustrated as to why you are not reaching your goal of ketosis. There are many keto specific phone apps out there. That is one assignment this month. Please find an app that suits your needs or at minimum start counting sugar.

My Experience and Benefits

I can attest to the fact that keto requires some adaptation time. Some positive effects I noticed immediately. Many took time. Once I broke through the first month, I really gained some great benefits. The first thing my husband and I noticed was increased mental acuity. The brain is a fatty organ. Fat coats the axons in the nerve cells to allow memory consolidation, better memory recall, and increased acetylcholine formation. Fat made our brains work better.

I had rapid waistline decreases from less bloating. Our faces slimmed down from less inflammation. Actual weight loss took a few months.

We experienced increased energy. Sometimes it almost felt excessive. We even felt like we had more time and vigor for life. Once we stabilized our blood sugar, and depended on stored fat for fuel, we were less dependent on food. We did not need to eat as often, which provided freedom from eating / cooking to do other things. We had more time to enjoy our evenings.

We also noticed more normal bowels. Not only does keto avoid most foot allergens that can cause irritable bowel, but the decrease in carbohydrate consumption also stabilizes gut flora.

Ketogenic Foods

To begin a ketogenic diet, you will need to prepare. That implies having a feasible eating routine. What you eat determines how quick you get into a ketosis state. The more prohibitive you are on your starches (under 15g every day), the quicker you will get to ketosis state.

Try not to Eat

- Sugar – nectar, agave, maple syrup, honey, etc.

- Grains – wheat, corn, rice, oats, etc.

- Starch/Tubers – potatoes, yams, beets, turnips, etc.

- Fruit – apples, bananas, oranges, etc.

You Can Eat

- Leafy Greens – spinach, kale, cabbage, collards, etc.

- Meats – Anything with fins, feathers, feet or eggs

- Above ground vegetables – broccoli, cauliflower, squash, etc.

- Nuts and seeds – macadamias, walnuts, sunflower seeds, almonds, etc.

- High Fat Dairy – hard cheeses, high fat cream, butter, etc.

- Avocado and berries – raspberries, blackberries, etc.

- Other fats – coconut oil, any nut oil, animal fats (bacon grease, duck fat, chicken fat, lard).

- Sweeteners – stevia, erythritol, and other low-carb sweeteners

- Liquids – apple cider vinegar, bulletproof coffee*, sea salt water, bone broth, collagen, protein powder, tea, lemon water

  o *bulletproof means adding a fat source to your coffee; you may use coconut cream, grass-fed butter, MCT oil, etc. This cuts down on the acidity of the coffee while providing extra brain fuel.

Areas of Dysfunction

Here are the top 10 reasons for failing this diet and how to avoid them. Actually, these are the top reasons for failing most diets.

1. No focus on quality

Be careful not just to eat bacon, cheese, and keto cookies. You still need to eat your vegetables and meats. Coffee is not a meal.

2. Feeling obligated to eat

If you are not hungry, you can wait until you are. When you become fat adapted, your appetite will change. Listen to when/what it wants. If you don't want dinner, you don't have to eat it.

3. Forgetting veggies

A ton of B vitamins are needed to break down fats with the oxidation cycle. Make sure you have at least 3 cups a day of greens or green drinks.

4. Too many "keto" treats, not enough food

Don't have your entire day's calories in just fat bombs and keto brownies.

5. Obsessed with tests

If your urine test strip doesn't say you are in ketosis, do not get discouraged. You will gain many benefits of this diet before it shows up on a test. Also, it takes a few days to weeks to get into measurable ketosis.

6.   Cheat meals or carb replenishing

As discussed earlier, high carbohydrate meals will make you sugar dependent again and knock you out of ketosis.

7.   Becoming a cheese-aholic

We discussed dairy for a whole chapter, it is not meant to be your main calorie source.

8.   Ignoring exercise or exercising too hard

Exercise will likely be difficult the first few weeks. Accept that you will not be hitting personal records for the beginning. Take more time for yoga and leisure exercise during this phase.

9.   Quitting to early-or going in too strong too fast without allowing adaptation

As stated, it takes a few days for some and a few weeks for others to hit ketosis. Do not get frustrated if you do not lose 10 lbs. in the first 2 weeks.

10. Treating it like an all or nothing deal

If you do fall off the bandwagon or realize you have been eating a no-no food for a while, do not quit. Learn from your mistakes and keep moving. Do not have one bite of cake and go eh, might as well eat the whole thing plus a pizza. Think about your vehicle for a moment. You do not just get a door ding and go eh, might as well total it.

How to Conquer the Drawbacks

You will likely notice body changes beside weight and not all of them are wonderful at first. Remember, we said this was an adaptation and forced adaptation is hard. How good you feel on keto the first few weeks is entirely dependent on your sugar dependency prior to starting. Here are some temporary negative side effects, how to combat them, and the reasons behind them.

Constipation-

Bowel changes can be due to eating less, consuming dairy, or dehydration. Some will use the restroom less due to less bulk of food consumed. Carbs are bulky. This is similar to how your dog poops more on cruddy dog food due to all the filler calories. Moral of the story, eat less means poop less. However, if the stool is difficult to pass you may need to drink more water, increase electrolyte consumption, or decrease dairy foods.

Weird Stool Consistency

Your stool may vary a great deal in the first few weeks. This can be due to yeast die off and a change in gut flora. It may be due to mucus formation from dairy. It could also be from your gallbladder trying to catch up to fat consumption, which causes your stool to float.

Sleep Changes

When your body is trying to increase your blood glucose, it uses adrenaline or Cortisol. Both of these are sleep inhibitive. They will likely wake you up a lot the first few weeks before becoming fat adapted. You will likely notice you require less sleep when you are fat adapted as well.

Acne or Rash

When you have a massive yeast die off in the body it often shows up as a rash. Increased hormone/Androgen production can also cause acne. You will likely have some hormone swings while your body is adapting.

Increases Trips to the Restroom

Sugar/Insulin makes you hold water weight. When you have less glucose and insulin, you hold less water. This means you pee, A LOT at first.

Keto Flu

This is another word for sugar withdrawal. Remember, to some people a sugar addiction is similar to cocaine. Some people have a morphine like addiction to grains and dairy. So when these individuals quit they can get shaky, sweaty, angry, dizzy, etc. Otherwise, this flu can be due to things like leaky gut and SIBO which we discussed a few chapters ago.

Food Shaming

You will need to become OK with asking the waitress to not bring the bread basket, no matter how many dirty looks you get. We are constantly brainwashed by the media as to what is healthy. There are so many things misleading us on our health conquering journey. So in order to overcome the innumerous odds that are stacked against you, it becomes necessary to change your philosophy. Once you change your mentality, saying no to the temptations around you, and finally reaching your goals becomes much more achievable.

You must learn to be OK with being called a "health nut," "granola eaters," or whatever other terms are out there. Take solace in the fact that you are different, so you will get different RESULTS than everyone else. Health efforts in this country are failing. In a decade of unlimited knowledge, people choose to ignore it. If you take the same path as everyone else you will end up like the majority end up with cancer, metabolic syndrome, or death.

Don't Succumb To Peer Pressure

It is ridiculous that in our society you are ridiculed for caring about your body. You only get one, it is your temple, worship it! That being said, if you live 100% strict on a protocol for 100% of your life then you will go bat shit crazy and have no friends. THERE IS A VERY PSYCHOLOGICAL ASPECT TO FOOD SO IT IS GOOD TO NOT MAKE YOURSELF FEEL LIKE A COMPLETE OUTSIDER 24/7. That being said, there are some changes that will be permanent and life-long but do not neglect to have fun or enjoy food. For example, some food allergies will require lifelong retraction, especially if they are driving an auto-immune disease like Celiac. These patients should never consume gluten again, however, they may still want a flourless chocolate cake on their birthday and that is fine! Just do not take it to the point where you are going completely backwards, binge drinking, eating processed foods, neglecting exercise, and eating fast food.

Saturday night is international cheat meal time, don't go past that. Don't eat a cheat meal so epic you ruin your progress. If you are 100% strict every day you have turned clean eating into an eating disorder. I think an 80/20 lifestyle is reasonable for most. Obviously there are times where 100 percent effort is needed, such as the first few weeks of keto. When on a strict protocol, stick to your guns. Do not be ashamed that your health in important to you. Shout it out loud that you are giving up crud to better yourself in the long run and that you will be done at x date and can regain festivities then. Once the intense period is over, eating strict 80% of the time and allowing fun 20% of the time is a much more sustainable mechanism for life. A quote I love is "Perfection is impossible. However, striving for perfection is not. Do the best that you can under the conditions that exist. That is what counts." –John Wooden

Assignments

Follow the Ketogenic Diet and count sugar consumption

Measure something besides your weight

Go out to dinner with friends and stick up for yourself. Do not ruin your progress because you feel self-conscious around your friends.

Month 11

Drugs, Core Work, and Seeking Help

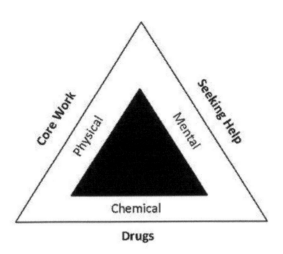

My Experience

I think I can speak for my genetics in saying that we are a group of do-it-yourself operators. Up to my early 20's I thought therapy, counseling, and hired help was a weakness. Lucky for me, I had a great doctor that encouraged me to balance out the mental side of my wellness. I started seeing the oddest Chiropractor I had ever met and I still could not describe what she did treatment wise but it freaking helped me. I still have not seen a psychiatrist per se but this woman was a chiropractic personal counselor/therapist if I had to give her a title. We talked about school stress, making big life decisions, insecurities, family relationships, intimate relationships, past hardships, etc. Then she would find exercises and treatments to help me.

Now, I have not had any kind of traumatic past or bad happenings in my life. I live a very blessed existence. This doctor still tremendously helped me in a time of turmoil. I was at a turning point in my career, my relationship, my location, and my family and couldn't handle the stress on my own. She empowered me to discover what I really wanted and map out how to get their without losing my mental health in the process. It is amazing how much talking to a professional can teach you about yourself.

I currently see a health coach to specifically focus on emotional help. She helps me with assignments, mindset, and emotional release to handle my stress more efficiently. I cry every time we speak and it's usually just from pure relief of unloading emotional tension. In the over-stimulating and busy world we live in, sometimes we just need help. The relief I get just from speaking to a professional of this kind is amazing. Words and consult are very powerful therapeutic tools.

Seeking Help

Getting help can be a medical necessity. We do not inherently know how to fix every problem or manage turmoil. Help can mean professional or just be from friends/family.

For certain situations, an unbiased ear is necessary. That is why I have a health coach. There are certain struggles I just want an outside opinion on. There are things I just don't think my family can be unbiased when giving advice. It is also easier to confess in an outside source because you have less fear of judgment.

In contrast, there are things your family is meant to help you with. It has been part of human culture forever to seek guidance from our elders and family. Moms are probably the most apt therapists in existence for most problems.

One assignment this month is to seek help from a professional. Who you see is completely personal preference. There are options including psychiatrist, health coach, Reike practitioner, NRT chiropractors, personal counselors, pastors, social workers, or psychologists. Find which fits your personal philosophies.

Day to Day Help

Of course, needing help goes beyond just medical needs. It can be discussed in regards to anything from school, moving, children, marriage, all the way to just getting daily chores done. I once asked a friend advice about hiring a house cleaner. Her words to me were:" I look forward to writing that check each month because it makes me so happy." If there are certain things on your to do list that stress you beyond belief, ask for help. Hire help. Delegate tasks. You do not have to do EVERYTHING.

Help=Freedom

I want you to start understanding that asking for help in your life only leads to more personal freedom. More personal freedom leads to happiness. This can be in regards to your schedule or just your overall mental health. The delegating tasks example is pretty self-explanatory as far as why it creates freedom in your week. However, let's talk about mental struggles for a second here. When you keep a problem to yourself it is a burden, when you share it with others, they carry a part of that burden. They share the load. It takes the weight off of your shoulders. It may not solve the problem at hand, but it will make you feel free. For example, a person coming out of the closet will feel more freedom. After years of carrying the secret of their sexuality, the truth really does set them free. It can apply to any mental struggle: marital problems, abuse, depression, not meeting preset standards of society, financial struggles, health maladies, etc. Keeping problems to yourself actually just hurts everyone around you. It leads to misunderstanding, grudges, communication error, and just overall misery for all parties involved. The truth is freedom. I have yet to meet someone with personal struggles that did not feel better when they finally came out about them. Seek help for your struggles. Talk to people. Shoving things under the rug helps no one. No matter how big or small the problem. Most fallouts in relationships of any kind are usually due to the words unsaid because the words were uncomfortable to let out; uncomfortable but necessary.

The Drug Talk

Now, with all this talk about mental health and seeking help from professionals we usually find a drug argument. Obviously, there are times when drugs are completely necessary. I have had a few suicides in my family that may have been prevented by proper pharmaceutical intervention. However, these drugs were not as widespread at that time. Both deaths occurred due to an inability to cope with an EXTREME trauma. Extreme trauma actually scars the brain; the brain is the slowest organ to heal. It takes YEARS.

So please do not take the following rant in the wrong way. I am not anti-drug. I am against over-prescribing and think it is a huge problem. I think we jump to quick fixes and do not take responsibility for our health by trying lifestyle changes first. I think that the pharmaceutical addiction has become an epidemic and is creating as many or more problems than it is curing. For example, painkillers are creating an opioid aka heroin epidemic. Do you think maybe we are overdoing it with the pain pills?

Your Drug May Be Your Problem

We are a pill popping country. The United States uses more prescriptions drugs that all other advanced civilizations combined. As a group, we tend to look for quick fixes and avoid treating the root cause of our problem: our lifestyle. We are sedentary, workaholic, overeating, sugar lovers. Usually, if these factors are addressed, there is no need for medication. Medication is meant to help your body on the way to recovery, but we all treat them as a crutch for our bad habits. By the way, most supplements are meant to do the same. Even we holistic individuals need to check ourselves at times. We cannot just switch medication addiction to supplement addiction. You should always be attempting to better yourself by identifying areas of weakness and trying to dominate them. The idea is to only be dependent on yourself, not some outside force to survive.

Our laziness is disturbing and needs to be addressed. Perhaps, by knowing the repercussions of our prescription addiction, we can change the direction we are headed. That direction is toward a bankrupt healthcare system due to overmedication and increased need for preventable emergency procedures.

Medication can be extremely harmful. Do not get me wrong, it is NEEDED in many situations. If you are about to die of infection in the hospital, medicate away. For example, my husband got kicked by a bull after trying to ride it and ended up septic in the ICU afterward. Medication and surgery very necessary. Of course this was technically a preventable disaster. A different lifestyle would have prevented this craziness, but you catch my drift. Medication is meant for unpreventable disasters. It is needed for situations where the risk of severe dysfunction is greater than the risk of ensuing a dangerous treatment. That risk assessment is an extremely personal decision. Let's look at rotator cuff surgery for example. A 20 year old athlete may find it worth getting it reattached. However, a 70 year old may not want to risk throwing a clot during surgery.

Some procedures/medication have very predictable risks. However, I would like to talk about some of the more ignored dangers of certain medication. Every drug commercial lists pages upon pages of possible side effects. Many of these are ignored either due to the wonderfully happy humans in the commercials running down a beach with their kids, or the "It will never happen to me" assumption. That is just plain stupid. I will admit, I used to have this mentality. I will still tell you, it's the equivalent of sticking your head up your ass. Obviously those side effects are listed because they DID happen to people. They are not just pulling things like vomiting and heart attack out of thin air. They happened to multiple test subjects or patients. Do not give me the "it's a one in a million chance" argument either. If it was only that likely, they would most likely have not linked the symptom to the particular drug. It had to happen to multiple people for them to make the correlation and can just as likely happen to you.

Now there are innumerable examples I can give you for drugs causing problems worse than the symptom you are using them for. Some of the first to mind are:

- Birth Control may lead to Infertility. The depo shot can cause this for up to 10 years!

- Anti-Depressants increase risk of suicide

- Estrogen replacement increases risk of stroke

- IBS drugs may cause violent diarrhea

- Just listen to the drug commercial

One of the most prescribed drugs in this country are Statins. These come with their own list of side effects. Let's delve into statins and use them as an in depth example of <u>why your drug may be your problem.</u> Typical drugs for heart disease do not prolong life, they just make the blood work look a bit better. Lifestyle changes are what prolong life.

Statins, Why Are They Prescribed?

Statins are commonly prescribed drugs used to treat high cholesterol. They work by blocking the enzyme that makes cholesterol in the body. Often people treated with statins respond well, and their cholesterol levels lower. Some of the most popular statin drugs are zocor, mevacor, lipitor, crestor and several others.

The majority of people using statin cholesterol-lowering drugs do so as they believe that lowering their cholesterol will prevent heart attacks and strokes. How many of these individuals do you think would continue to take these drugs if they knew that their drugs had been linked to increased risk of heart attack and increased risk of stroke? Probably no one. In fact, there is no evidence that these drugs prolong life. That is because lifestyle kills you. You were not born with a statin deficiency. Your body was designed perfectly. We just like to attempt to destroy our actually protective physiology.

A cholesterol level of 200 is not very dangerous to your health. It can cause serious health implications only when it rises above 400. But modern health professionals blindly make you a "good" candidate for statin drugs as soon as your cholesterol level goes above 200. The pharmaceutical companies keep pushing for lower cholesterol limits to create more dependant patients. Not so long ago 300 was the standard. They are now trying to get the standard below 200. I would like to point out that cholesterol below 150 is actually dangerous for your brain and unabashedly leads to depression and alzheimers-like symptoms. That is not to mention the muscle pain produced as well.

Elevated cholesterol may be easily controlled by putting you on a low glycemic diet. You can totally avoid statin drugs by engaging in regular exercise and adding more fiber to your diet. As discussed in the sugar chapter, high cholesterol is usually due to just plain overeating, especially sugar intake.

What is Cholesterol and what does it do?

Cholesterol is vital for life. It creates hormones, cell membranes, nerve lining, and feel good hormones(neurotransmitters). People deficient in cholesterol will experience memory loss, pain, low to no sex drive, clumsiness, poor brain function, and decreased healing capacity.

Cholesterol is a waxy substance used for wound healing. I like to call cholesterol natures band-aid. When there is an injury, the liver makes more cholesterol to help patch it up. About 50% of this comes from liver, and 50% from diet. That is why people can eat low fat and still have high cholesterol. The liver will make it when needed. Drugs will interfere with this process.

When there is an injury, infection or trauma cholesterol will increase. Even if you have a cold/flu it can temporarily increase your blood work numbers. That is the body doing its job. Where the problem lies is in artery blockage. Artery blockage can lead to stroke, heart attack, blood clots, etc. Why would the body clog up an artery? It goes back to the band-aid analogy. When the artery lining is injured by things like inflammation from poor diet choices cholesterol comes in to be the band-aid to the injury. Then we keep eating fast food and keep injuring the lining with inflammation and the body keeps putting on more band-aids until eventually blood flow cannot get through. The band-aid created a traffic jam. Let's say blood cells are like semi trucks. Semi truck cannot get through the jam. So we create motorcycles instead by taking blood thinners. It thins the blood so it can get through. Not that it really shrinks the cell but I think you get the picture.

So you probably notice that the root cause of the problem is the inflammation we have discussed so often in this book. Now I hope you realize the implications of taking hold or your diet and lifestyle so that you do not need to be drug dependant later on. How to know if you are inflamed? The test usually used to determine if you have chronic inflammation is a C-reactive protein (CRP) blood test. CRP level is used as a marker of inflammation in your arteries. There are a number of blood work markers that can be taken to test inflammation. If course if you have things like chronic pain, high cholesterol, poor brain function, etc that is pretty indicative.

Statins Increase Pain

Human research has also linked statin use to muscle injury which includes back pain. Most physicians now agree that statins can indeed cause muscle pain and weakness in some people. The side effects most commonly associated with statin use involve muscle cramping, soreness, fatigue, weakness, and, in rare cases, rapid muscle breakdown that can lead to death. These occur in 60% of those taking the drug. You see, everyone assumes side effects only happen to one of every few thousand people and that is simply not the case. Of course, there are many reasons for back pain. The main cause is a weak core.

Core Strength

When I use the word core, most people's minds go immediately to the 6-pack abs picture in their mind. I am here to tell you that is false. There are many athletes and bodybuilders with sexy abs that still blow their back out regularly. The washboard abs are not the picture of health we once thought. People that focus too much on this area are actually more likely to become injured.

The area of the body, which is commonly referred to as the core, is your midsection and it involves all your muscles in that area including the front, back and sides. The core includes the traverse abdominals (TVA), erector spinal, obliques, diaphragm, glutes, pelvic floor, and your lower lats. These muscles work as stabilizers for the entire body. They form the shape of a cylinder around your abdomen and have to all work in conjunction to keep you breathing and keep your spine safe.

If any of these core muscles are weakened, it could result in lower back pain or protruding waistlines. Keeping these core muscles strong can do wonders for your posture and help give you more strength in other exercises like running and walking.

Fashion Fads Ruin Abs

So where did things go wrong? Why do we breathe incorrectly? It seems like a pretty innate thing right? Well guess what, most babies and children do breath correctly at first. Then we put them in from of the TV all day and they develop rolled forward shoulders that crushed the diaphragm and digestive organs and we wonder why they develop asthma and indigestion. Then many of us have office jobs and sit eight to nine hours a day. Add another hour or two of driving time, and that adds up to a lot of sitting. Prolonged sitting and no exercise weakens the muscles of your midsection. Also, with most females, we are taught to suck it in. Stand up straight and tuck in our bellies. Womens physiology is constantly being bombarded by societal expectation. From the corset generations to 4 inch heels there has always been something there to destroy our core and low back strength. Let's talk about physiology vs. glamour for a moment. A small waist leads to a weak spine. Now I am not saying that fat is healthy or that you should be round. Your waist to hip ratio is supposed to be around 0.8. However, expansion is more stable than "sucking it in."

Abdominal Bracing/Breathing

Most responsible patients ask what they can do at home to prevent pain or spinal injury. Abdominal activation exercises will help any condition from indigestion, hiatal hernia, low back pain, rib pain, shallow breathing, all the way to successfully getting through natural labor. Proper breathing is like a massage to your internal organs.

The first step is to learn abdominal bracing. I want you right now to touch your belly between your hip and belly-button. Apply pressure. Now cough, laugh, clear your throat, or push down like you have to poo. That flexing of abdominal muscle is bracing. You innately do this during the aforementioned tasks. The trick is to practice doing it on cue. Ever notice how people grunt when lifting heavy? It's not just to be obnoxious, its because it activates the core. Bracing during any exercise or daily chore is the most important exercise to protect your spine.

Proper Breathing

The most important thing to know about breathing is that your stomach should expand (look fatter) as you breath in. This expansion is what brings in more air, takes pressure off of the neck and upper back, and protects the low back.

Try this: take a deep breath in while looking at a mirror. Did your shoulders move? Did they come up to reach your ears? THAT IS INCORRECT! If your shoulders move a lot in breathing, it creates too much rib movement. This can create recurring rib pain, upper Trapezius pain, as well as hiatal hernias. If you do this breathing during a heavy lift, you will throw out your back. So how do we avoid the back issues when lifting couches or just your grandkids?

Once you can get the bracing activation under you fingers as we practiced, we need to add deep breathing. So, when the ab muscles brace, keep them braced and try to inhale and make your hand move up with your belly. For a better visual representation of this watch videos about DNS (Dynamic Neuromuscular Stabilization), a common physical therapy technique. Or just watch a baby breath. They have nice round bellies that go up and out when they inhale. Making sure your stomach moved more than your ribs when breathing helps digestion, moves the bowels, increases lung capacity, makes athletics easier, and mobilizes the spine. Look at strongman competitors. They ALWAYS have very round bellies. However, they often are not fat. Why? It is because they are masters at abdominal breathing and core activation. That is why they can lift a truck without hurting their back. We all need to remember this in our daily lives. When we lift something heavy, we should be bracing our guts as if we were about to get punched. If I were winding up to hit you, you wouldn't "suck it in" right? The suck in your gut attitude is harmful to our backs. If I were to wind up to sock you in the gut, you would brace it as hard as you can. You would bear down and hold your breath right? That is because that is what is protective to the spine and organs.

Some safe core exercises are planks, v-sits, elevated leg holds, yoga, isometric holds, and bracing during weight bearing exercise. Traditional Sit Ups are actually bad. I have one uncle who significantly reduced his back pain by avoiding this exercise. He was a Marine and had been doing a zillion of them for years.

Our core is meant to be active during every minute of our lives. Therefore, longer holds are more beneficial for retraining it. It should also be exercised during any physical activity. You noticed I said weight bearing exercise? There are days my abs are sorer from squats than from v-ups. That is because when I am hitting a heavy weight, I have to activate my abdominal wall extremely hard to stay stable. My abs also get sore from running because I am keeping them active to keep my hips and back in place. You could work your abs sufficiently without doing any "abs" exercises. You need only to keep them active during your daily exercise routine.

Assignments

Evaluate your Prescription Cabinet and identify lifestyle factors you can change to reduce dependency

Seek help from professionals. This can be for any goal or symptom, healthcare related or not.

Practice Abdominal Breathing/Bracing. Watch a DNS video for more help on exercises

Month 12

Intermittent Fasting, Acupuncture, and Personal Development

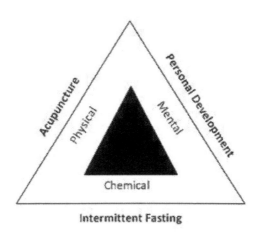

Intermittent Fasting

My Experience

The topics in this chapter are not last because they have any less efficacy than other chapters. I simply presented this book in an order similar to the sequence of health changes I have implemented in my life. Most topics I discovered either through other medical professionals, my experience, or personal development.

Acupuncture is a recent love of mine because it helps me when I feel like I just have pain all over and am falling apart due to stress. It gets my stomach relaxed and regulates digestion. My husband goes for acupuncture every time his sleep gets out of whack or if he starts getting night sweats. It has been a great addition to our health routine. As I have said previously, I would like to think that my profession can fix anything. However, some patients respond to certain treatments and others do not.

Acupuncture addresses things for me that chiropractic and massage do not. It treats a different element of our systems.

Acupuncture

There are many explanations for how and why acupuncture works. I would like to share with you the reason that makes the most sense to me. Our bodies are made up of electromagnetic fields. That is why an MRI (Magnetic Resonance Imaging) works, it is a giant magnet that detects changes in energy. Specifically it detects the protons released from hydrogen atoms from the water we are composed of. You can think of a magnetic field like a circuit of electricity. There has to be a fully connected circle or the energy flow does not work. Electricity in the body is called Chi. Acupuncture optimizes the flow of chi. If your chi is blocked in an area, there is a break in the electromagnetic circuit. Acupuncture will use needles or other stimulating mechanisms to reconnect this circuit. Since this chi flows throughout all our bodily systems, acupuncture has implications in the management of any medical condition. I always get asked what to see an acupuncturist for and the answer is really ANYTHING. Other countries use acupuncturists as their primary physician because they are trained to address any condition. Now, I am not saying to seek one out for emergency situations by any means. However, I see my acupuncturist for anything from digestive problems, knee pain, periods cramps, to acne.

What to expect

Acupuncturists diagnose chi deficiencies by looking at a series of key points in your body as well as your symptoms. Each visit you will be evaluated based on your tongue, pulses, muscle tonicity, presents symptoms, etc. Based on the findings from this, your acupuncturist will needle you for certain patterns of dysfunction in order to restore chi. it can be aimed at any goal. Your goal may be pain relief, fertility, digestive aid, sleep aid, bladder function, sexual function, brain clarity, and many more. Your goals will dictate the treatment. It is not a one size fits all approach. It is based on your body at that time that day.

The Needles

Many are afraid of needles. An acupuncture needle is not the size of thing that you would use for a vaccination. The needle is about the size of a human hair. It is very thin and more often than not you cannot feel them. Occasionally, a really active point may sting a bit. The pain is far less than even getting numbed at the dentist. If you have an extreme needle aversion, there are other things used to stimulate points such as cupping, magnets, electrical stimulation, heat lamps, Chinese medical massage, acupressure, etc.

Is it safe?

Anytime you wonder if a therapy is safe or not, think about how much the doctor pays in malpractice. Chiropractors and Acupuncturists pay less than $5,000 a year in malpractice. Your typical medical doctor has $500,000 to $1,000,000 a year in malpractice insurance. So which do you think has less incidence of injury? The truth is in most parts of the body you could put an acupuncture needle in a few inches without injuring anything. The only areas of concern are over the torso and lungs.

History

Acupuncture has been a part of Chinese Medicine for 2,500 years. The fact that we see this treatment as "alternative" is almost sad as the practice has been around and effective for so long. In fact, it is still the primary form of care in many eastern countries. The medicine we use for primary care in the U.S. is only a few hundred years old. When you consider how long the technique has served patients, it should not be questioned as a viable healthcare preference.

There are many legendary health practices that have long since been ignored. Let's move into another age-old health technique, intermittent fasting.

Intermittent Fasting

Intermittent fasting is a new technique for my household as well. It was a complete paradigm shift for me after being on adrenal fatigue protocols for most of grad school that required constant calorie input. I was eating all day every day. It was kind of exhausting. Learning about fasting gave me the confidence to try something new. I was more than impressed when I had more energy instead of sugar crashing hard as I had expected. Altering the timing of my food intake helped with energy, sleep, digestion, weight, bloating, and productivity. I did/do the 16-8 style of fasting discussed in this chapter.

Intermittent fasting is used to describe a period of dieting that alternates between periods of fasting and periods of eating food regularly. There is actually a reason behind that. Humans have reportedly fasted ever since their existence. The reasons were simple--the food was scarce in certain periods e.g. winter time and in some nations and religions like Christianity and Islam, fasting became the norm.

We are all culturally wired to consume our food during certain times of the day e.g. breakfast at 9, lunch at 1 pm, and dinner at 8pm. The truth of the matter is, there is much controversy surrounding the subject about when we should consume certain meals to facilitate weight loss and health and when we shouldn't. The typical pattern of 3 meals a day and a large dinner is only making us fatter. So let's look at why IF may be a smart alternative.

Reasons Intermittent Fasting Works

Eat when the sun is out:

Your metabolism and circadian rhythm are attached to the light dark cycle. When the sun is out, we burn more calories. This is one reason we fatten up in the winter: less sun equals slower metabolism. On way to focus your fasting is around darkness. That way you are not eating calories when they are not needed. Many will get weight loss benefits from eating on this schedule alone. Do not eat in the dark.

The Sugar/Fatty Acid cycle:

It is simple; if sugar is present the body will use it for fuel. If sugar is not present, we will switch to fat for fuel. Fat fuel will be taken from your own tissue when dietary fuel is not present. The only caveat to this is excess Cortisol secretion will cause you to use muscle tissue for energy. That is why people in extreme stress will not eat and waste their muscle away. So, if you start fasting and notice your muscle mass depleting, you may need to investigate your life stressors more thoroughly.

Evolution:

Our hunter-gatherer ancestors did not have constant food availability. In fact, food was not readily available until the advent of refrigerators and grocery stores. For most of human history we fasted for long periods between meals. In hunter gatherer times this may have been days. Once we started farming this time grew less and less. Our bodies are rigged for fasting. We were not meant to depend on six small meals a day. This may be advantageous for treating certain conditions at first, but really our metabolism is equipped for long periods without food. We are only so dependent on snacking now due to blood sugar instabilities and hormone imbalances. It is beneficial to address these imbalances before starting IF. That is why I waited to talk about this until later chapters. Remember, you are supposed to follow the book in order to avoid any crazy withdrawal symptoms and fix physiology first.

Advantages of fasting:

-Reduced amount of body fat

-Reduced blood sugar levels

-Reduced amounts of insulin and insulin resistance

-Accelerated fat burning and fat oxidation

-Raised levels of Growth Hormone

-Reduced stress related from food

-Reduced chronic inflammation

This looks awesome right? Let's take a closer look on how fasting helps and affects our bodies in 6 different ways:

No 1: Insulin reduction. Remember insulin is released to bring blood sugar down.

When you eat (especially sugar), insulin levels start to rise up in anticipation of glucose intake. Without this fat storage hormone around, we are more likely to use our own stores for fuel.

No 2: Controls blood sugar. Blood sugar (glucose) is the level of sugar found in our blood. When we consume excessive amounts of food, our systems go on overload trying to catch up with the sudden rises and repeat supply of sugar. It is hard to lose weight with an overabundance of easy fuel present in the blood. We are hard wired to store this fuel source as fat for later use in fasting periods that never come in today's paradigm.

Fasting fact: Even periods of short fasting e.g. 12 hours, enable our systems to control blood glucose. The "low sugar" condition isn't as frequent as many people think. It takes a medical check-up to be diagnosed and it's called "hypoglycemia". Studies conducted on the impact of fasting and blood sugar levels demonstrated that blood sugar didn't drop below normal. Thus, most folks who assume they have a low sugar episode or syndrome are actually not. Most people that assume they are hypoglycemic are actually just experiencing sugar withdrawal from their previous high carbohydrate meal. Remember, sugar is like cocaine to the brain so withdrawals can be severe.

No 3: Stimulates fat burning. With a lack of food calories, fatty acids are freed and circulate through the bloodstream to be used as energy sources by your muscle tissue and vital organs. Fasting here enables the system to take a break from depositing fat and burn this fat instead for energy! Fat burn is the highest between 8 and 30 hours after a meal, so no need to fast for longer periods of time (unless doing SIBO protocol in earlier chapters).

Fasting tip: If you fast between 12-14 hours, you will start triggering fat burning as your main energy source. It is commonly said that your burn calories while you sleep. The main reason for this is that you are fasting while you sleep so your body has to burn its own fat for energy. Eating too late at night will make you miss this mechanism.

No 4: Raises Growth Hormone (GH) levels. Fasting also stimulates Growth Hormone release especially when combined with working out and healthy sleep patterns. GH is at its peak during your teenage years (this perhaps explains why most of us have gone through the "bottomless pit" situation). The nice thing about Growth Hormone is that it helps enhance muscle volume, that way you should not lose muscle mass during IF.

No 5: Reduces inflammation. Without chronic insulin release, there are less inflammatory mechanisms activated during IF. Also, being less overweight decreases inflammation. A University of Utah study has found that individuals who fasted even for one day per month, had 40% less risk to experience clogged arteries as opposed to those that didn't fast.

No 6: Triggers rejuvenation and cleansing on a cellular level. When you are not busy digesting all the time, you allow the body the energy for detoxification. The process of cellular cleansing from junk has caught the attention of cancer researchers who see it as a potential treatment for cancer. Researchers have shown that fasting 2x a week could reduce the risk of developing Alzheimer's and Parkinson's disease. In simple words, fasting triggers the death of already damaged and weak immune cells and when the system goes through such a transitional back-up stage, it produces new healthier cells.

IF and The Brain

Diet habits and changes have been found to bear a strong impact on brain function. Kids suffering from epileptic episodes experience them less when fasting or following calorie restriction diets. It is estimated that fasting helps trigger protective functions which help control the over-stimulated brain signals of epileptic patients. Some children have also shown some improvement from following a high fat and low carb diet (e.g. Ketogenic diet). But it's not just epileptic brains who experience over-stimulation. Normal/average brains can also experience another form of imbalance and over-excitement which affects brain focus and function, when they are being overfed. Overeating is overstimulation.

Typical Question/Concerns about IF

No 1: What about breakfast?

We typically encourage patients to eat breakfast because they are caffeine addicts all morning and binge eat later in the evening. Caffeine inhibits appetite at first but stimulates metabolism to make you hungry later. This becomes a problem because people binge on high carbohydrate and sugary foods once their caffeine wears off. This is a weight gain pattern of behavior. If people eat a high protein/fat meal earlier in the day, they tend to not have these cravings at night. If you are in a ketogenic balance and intermittent fasting, the evening carbohydrate cravings tend not to be an issue. Once your body adapts to intermittent fasting and/or keto, you will be satisfied without all the treats. Your body will be more efficient at creating its own energy and you will hence be less dependent on stereotypical eating patterns such as breakfast. However, if this is your favorite meal or if you are in high amounts of activity in the AM, you may want to bias your fasting so that you can include breakfast. For example, I do Crossfit at 6AM so I fast later in the evening.

No 2: What happens with starvation mode?

Intermittent fasting done correctly should not be starvation mode. It is not a severe calorie reduction diet. It is simply altering the time and frequency that you eat. You may notice you eat less calories than you did before because your body is more efficient at producing energy and less dependent on constant caloric intake for fuel. Starvation mode occurs when your weekly caloric intake is at a 5,000, or perhaps even higher, deficit from your caloric burn. For example: if your weekly calories come out to 700 calories a day, you may be in starvation mode. However, if your cal/day are still above 1,200-2,00 (depending on body type), you will not enter this mode.

No 3: What about fueling the metabolic fire?

The answer is, you are fueling the fire. IF should be done with food lifestyles such as Paleo and Keto. Remember, Fat are logs, protein is kindling, and carbohydrates are the paper. If you put logs on the fire, it will burn for days.

No 4: What if I'm hungry?

This is normal at the very beginning but as we discussed previously, switching your eating patterns is not an overnight process as you need plenty of time, patience, and practice to make it through. You have to remember that you are trying to reset your circadian rhythm here. During the first few days of IF, you may feel hungry during the hours you used to eat previously—after all, you may have followed the same eating pattern for years so change isn't easy. The initial days of IF may feel kind of uncomfortable, as other members have told us but if you are patient enough, your system will get used to it and IF will become a habit. You will be really compensated for your effort. Full adaptation can take 1-3 months depending on your diligence, so do not quit on week 2.

No 5: My exercise capacity sucks.

This is a temporary feeling during adaptation. Once you learn to use fat for fuel, your athletic ability should return. It should improve in the long run because your body will know how to perform without carbohydrate constantly being fed to the muscle.

Intermittent Fasting Plans:

There are many ways to implement fasting. Choose the plan that fits your lifestyle.

EAT-STOP-EAT (fast for 24 hours once or twice a week).

It's hard to talk about 24-hour fasting windows without giving credit to Brad Pilon and his writing piece "EAT-STOP-EAT." The regime calls for 1-2 24-hour fasting periods per week, on the days that suit your daily schedule.

2 to 5 diet: (five days of typical eating and 2 days of eating low calories).

The 5:2 IF pattern calls for eating as usual for 5 days in a week, and fasting for the remaining 2 days of the week (taking only 500 calories). The protocol considers the evidence of IF paired with an eating plan that is low in calories to allow weight loss without starvation. This plan offers a very nutritionally stabilized intake, and it easily becomes a part of most schedules as it lets you choose the two days you are going to fast/eat less amount of calories.

There was one study with 100 female subjects split into 2 groups. One group consumed 25% less calories every day, while the other group was following the 5:2 fasting pattern, fasting for 2 days of the week only. While both of these groups eventually lost weight after a period of 6 months following these plans, the female group following the 5:2 diet lost more fat around the belly region and also showed more balanced blood sugar levels.

16-8 IF plan (16 hours of fasting-8 hours eating normally).

Also called "the lean gains method", the 16/8 IF plan is probably the most popular. This IF method became famous by Martin Berkhan who initiated the "lean gains" act. This encourages a 16-hour fasting window, followed by 8 hours eating normally. This is a highly versatile IF plan and again, you can choose which 16 hours you'll be fasting, and which 8 hours you'll be eating normally. Most people though choose sleeping hours to cover their 16 hour fasting period and eat normally between 11am-7pm. This is probably the best plan for intense athletes. It is my preference, although I prefer breakfast hours.

Warrior mode: (20 hours of fasting window/4 hours of eating).

The warrior style mode calls for fasting for 20 consecutive hours and eating only 4, usually at dinnertime. So all your day calories you will need for the day, will be taken during that 3-5 dinnertime period. This is one of the most aggressive IF methods, many of those that tried this reported saving huge amounts of valuable time.

Meal Prepping

Planning ahead is the only way to be successful with restrictive diets. We do meal prep Sundays at my house. We defrost a bunch of meat. Roast up all the veggies. Make soups and crock pot meals. That way we have food pre-made all week. It is a lot easier to stay on track when all you need to do is reheat.

Another key tool for success of any kind is personal development. It is a way to acquire knowledge that helps you reach your goals; which is something you are already starting by reading this book.

Personal Development

Many have an unfounded belief about self-help books. It is not a weakness to diagnose your shortcomings and work on them. It is not a weakness to get amped up about life. It is also not a weakness to identify goals and figure out how to accomplish them. It is in fact strength, and a quality of winners, to try and better yourself every day. Just because you exist a certain way right now, does not mean that has to be your reality forever. The average CEO reads 60 books a year.

Personal Development can encompass many realms. It can apply to anything from personality, relationships, athletics, career, motivation, nutrition, health, to parenting. You can learn about these topics from podcasts, books, radio, professionals, blogs, YouTube videos, social media, or just from your elders. The point is to seek out these things to better yourself, and to not feel self-conscious in doing so. Remember, if you are not building momentum forward in your life, you are likely going backwards. You should do something to improve yourself every day.

Podcasts are a recent obsession in our life. We follow the groups that serve our self-interest. For example, we listen to one called Barbell Shrugged that is all about Crossfit, exercise, nutrition, and winning at life. I listen to media about mindset, social media marketing, functional medicine, nutrition, relationships, career women, etc. I find that podcasts and similar media help me focus. They spur "ah ha" moments, motivate me, and help me create plans of action. I think finding the right speakers can really help you focus to reach any goal. I listen to one called The MFCEO Project. It helps me learn how to be a better entrepreneur and how to keep momentum.

Power List

One great technique to start a self-improvement journey is called a power list. I learned this form the aforementioned podcast. Here is how to create this list. Think about a goal. Let's use weight loss as an example. Say you want to lose 20 pounds. If this is the case, your power list should consist of steps to reach that goal. Choose 5 or less things for your daily list. For weight loss, number one and two on your list should be exercise 20 minutes and hit a 500 calorie deficit. Maybe another goal is to finish a book, so number 3 should be read one chapter a day. Starting to make sense?

The power list is 5 things a day that are an action plan to reach your goal. A goal without an action plan is a wish. There is no magic fairy that is going to grant your wishes. If you finish your five small things each day, you win the day. If you do your list all week, you win the week. Eventually you win the year. You lose those 20 pounds.

This method can obviously be used for any goal, not just weight. It can be used for money making goals, any self-improvement, or even relationship help. You goal may be for a better relationship with your spouse. Then your number 1 action step each day may be 30 minutes of no technology time with your significant other each day. If your goal is to squat 300 pounds, your number 1 may be to do leg exercises each day. Think about this, just because you want to lift 300 pounds and lift every day, doesn't mean you will reach your goal in one month. It may take a year to hit that weight. Remember this concept with your other goals. You can reach anything you want to achieve. Sometimes the ignored factor is time. A 300 pound personal record may take a year or more as may your weight loss or other goals. Take things one day at a time and win your power list so that you do not get overwhelmed by this timeline.

Moral of the story, don't quit on yourself or your relationships. I see it as a sign of strength to try counseling books or therapists to work on quality of life. It means you are not a quitter. It means you will not let your setbacks or inefficiencies hold you down. Hiding from problems doesn't help anyone involved in your life. If you feel lost or like you don't have a plan to reach your goal, start with the power list.

Assignments

Create a Power List of 5 things to finish each day this month

Try one of the Intermittent Fasting Patterns

Try Acupuncture

Bonus Month

Balancing Macros, Squats, and Sleep

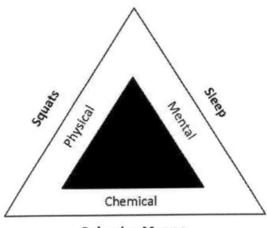

Balancing Macros

My Experience

I am a terrible sleeper. Nights that I do not wake up at least once are in the minority. It is a constant struggle to control. I used to lay wide awake until 2AM and then never want to wake up. That or I woke up at 2AM unable to fall back asleep. I have been an inconsistent sleeper since childhood. Even my mom remembers me terrifying her in the middle of the night just standing in her doorway because I was awake but not quite coherent.

Since working on things in this book such as digestion, blood sugar, and intermittent fasting I have drastically improved my sleep efficiency. The things that help me with sleep the best are balancing macros and morning exercise. I have a number of patients that agree when they increase their protein, their sleep and energy improve. It simple, when you give the body the nutrients and movement it requires, it will repay you positively.

I was listening to one athlete that had over 90% sleep efficiency according to her fitness tracker. This means that almost every minute she spends in bed she is actually sleeping, not tossing and turning. Most people are much lower than this on efficiency. When asked how she gets her sleep, she simply stated "she is flipping exhausted from her exercise routine." Getting your body enough movement is key. You can also bet that this particular Crossfit athlete was hitting her macros.

Balancing Macros

While I know I said that Paleo is the best option for a lifelong maintenance diet, there is still a lot of room for error. For example, you can say you are "Paleo" and still eat maple syrup treats and fruit all day. The best way to stay on track, eat what you want and still keep a healthy life with optimal performance is to balance macros. Balancing macros can be applied to any lifestyle whether Paleo, vegan, gluten free, etc.

This type of an eating pattern is popular with bodybuilders and athletes because it lowers body fat percentages while keeping optimal athletics. However, it can be applied for the average Joe as well. You do not need to have a goal of 10% body fat to benefit from the principals here. A macro diet means hitting proper proportions of the three core nutrients.

There are three **macro**nutrients: carbohydrate, fat, and protein. See the list below for some healthy examples of each. A more complete list (including junk food) is listed in the appendix. However, most junk food may be considered a carbohydrate.

Protein	Carbohydrate		Fat	
Meat:	Veggies:	Fruit:	Healthy Fats	Omega 3's
Anything that has **Feathers, Fins,** or **Feet**...and eggs. When possible choose **organic chicken, wild fish**, and **grass fed beef.** 1 serving: the size and thickness of your palm.	Broccoli Asparagus Spinach squash Kale Romaine lettuce Cucumber Bell peppers Celery Zucchini Cucumber Carrots	Green Apples Berries Grapefruit Pears Plums Cantaloupe Orange Melon	Avocado Coconut oil Nut oils Olive oil Olives Eggs Animal fat Bone broth	Flaxseed/oil Salmon Grass fed beef Chia seeds Walnuts Omega 3 rich eggs

Typically, these nutrients are encouraged to be consumed in 40:30:30 ratios. That is 40% carbohydrates, 30% protein, and 30% fat. As with most things in this book though, I encourage you to find which ratio is best for your body. I work best at 20-25% carbohydrates, 25% protein, and 50% fat. My husband requires more carbohydrates than that. We are all different. Your macronutrient needs depend on genetics, athletic inclinations, gut health, and goals. For example, your ratios will be different if you are trying to build muscle vs. lean out.

As a reminder, Ketogenic diet is a modification in macronutrient ratios. It consists of 70% fat, 20% protein, and 10% carbohydrate. Diets for muscle gain are 55% carbohydrates, 30% protein, and 15% fat. Paleo would typically be 40% fat, 25% carbohydrate, and 35% protein. The standard American recommendations are 55% carbohydrate, 15% protein, and 30% fat. Atkins would be about 50% protein, 35% fat and 15% carbohydrate. So you can see how each person can choose different ratios based on their overall goals.

Measuring

The most dedicated way to measure macros is to purchase a scale and weigh your proteins, measure out your fats per teaspoon and carbs per cup. Then log these into a food journal or bodybuilding app on your phone. However, this can get rather overbearing. It is great to do this method for a few weeks just to get the hang of portion sizes, but unless you have that 10% body fat goal it is not necessary to do this long term.

I think the easiest way to measure macros is by designing your plate in the following manner. Half of your plate should be vegetables, a quarter can be a starch or fruit, and a quarter should be protein. Fat is generally drizzled on top of all of these for flavor. Use the picture below to create your plate.

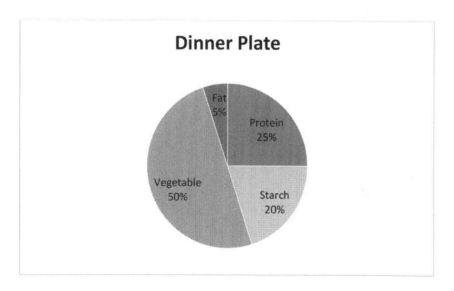

The importance of measuring is dependent on your body composition goals. The more exact you are the better results you will get. For me, the most dependable way to lose weight was with a Fitbit. Any of the athletic watches will track calories burned. You can also log the food you ate that day with portion sizes. It will also track your macros. With the knowledge of how many calories you actually burn per day, you can more accurately make caloric goals for eating. For weight loss that doesn't deplete you, you want to shoot for a 500 calorie a day deficit. If you have a 1,000 calorie deficit at the end of the day, you will hit starvation mode, feel trashy, and likely not lose weight. The fit watches are great for showing people how many calories their body actually needs to function. Very few of us accurately predict our caloric need. Most people go by the 2,000 calorie a day standard. Most women assume 1,200 a day is sufficient for weight loss. We forget that we all have different weights, muscle mass, and activity levels. These factors together determine caloric need.

There are some calculators available to figure out your basal metabolic rate (the rate you burn calories at rest). However, most do not account for activity level. There are some other calculators that include activity estimates. However, activity trackers (such as Fitbit) are much more accurate. For me, most calculators would say I need 1,700 calories a day. Now this is pretty close to correct. However, with my watch I see that on active days I can burn up to 3,000. So you can see how if on a 3,000 cal day, if I only ate 1,700 or the stereotypical 1,200, I would be pretty tired and miserable.

Fatigue

I will say with utmost confidence that most fatigue is due to insufficient calories/nutrients or unbalanced macros. A carbohydrate only diet leads to fatigue and muscle wasting. Insufficient fat leads to brain disorders like depression. Insufficient protein leads to fatigue and weakness. Lack of vegetables leads to pretty much any negative symptom. I would bet that if you start tracking macros and calories, without even changing food quality, you will notice a difference in energy. FOOD IS FUEL. If you put gas in the vehicle, it will run. It can be that simple. You don't have to have a diagnosable disease to have fatigue. It can just be insufficient nutrients. This is especially true for moms. Many mothers will spend so much time and effort keeping their families fed that they do not eat. I hear it over and over. They cook dinner and do not eat it. Then they barely get sleep on top of that and they are fatigued. Eventually this leads to adrenal problems and vertigo. The answer to all this; eat the calories your body needs! Do not fuel with only caffeine. Balance your macros.

Another fun fact, most people will sleep better when they have sufficient nutrients as well. Most sleep problems are driven by surges in Adrenaline or Cortisol. These hormones are trying to bring up your blood sugar for energy. If you have food for energy, there is no need to surge adrenaline. Carbohydrate only diets will destroy a circadian rhythm with these Cortisol surges. Cortisol inhibits melatonin. If you have tried melatonin and it did nothing, you are producing too much Cortisol! The number 1 way to address this is to change the diet.

Sleep Hygiene

Here is a quick note on getting better sleep. As we stated, the most important thing is to avoid surges in adrenaline. Adrenaline and Cortisol being high in the evening keeps your mind racing and make it hard to fall asleep until past midnight. Random spikes throughout the night are what wakes you up startled. The number one thing causing unexpected adrenaline or Cortisol spikes in low blood sugar. Number two is acute stress like family or job problems. The blood sugar chapter goes into depth on how to avoid this happening but what it really comes down to is eating less sugar and avoiding 100% carbohydrate meals. The main foods that can cause stimulant releases throughout the night are alcohol, sweets, popcorn, ice cream, cereal, etc. Avoid these high glycemic foods and stick to the protein later in the evening.

On the other hand, some people may have a hard time sleeping if they eat too large of a meal late at night. This is due to digestion inhibiting sleep. If you eat, your metabolism increases which makes you hotter. A revved up metabolism makes that body ready to do activity and burn calories. Be sure to eat dinner 3-4 hours before bed to avoid this phenomenon. You want to signal the body that you are cooling down and relaxing. Your metabolism should be slowing down for sleep.

I know there are a few of you arguing right now saying that large meal helps you fall asleep. Be careful with this, a large meal will raise your blood sugar so that you are sleepy. However, it will subsequently drop it leading to those adrenaline surges at 2-3AM. You need to be done digesting your food before bed if you expect to hit REM sleep and get good restorative rest.

Other stimulants to avoid after dinner for optimal sleep are intense TV shows, exercise, work, or any project that gets you too amped up. Stop for a moment and think about the struggle of putting kids to bed. When putting kids to bed you have to read to them and lay with them quietly for a while before they can wind down for bed. If they are running around the house playing tag and eating cookies it's hard to get them to sleep right? Adults are wired the same way. Stop treating yourself worse than the kids. Create your own bedtime ritual. An hour before bed read a book, do some stretching, do a puzzle, watch animal planet...well these are some of my personal examples anyways. Do something to help you unwind.

As far as exercise goes, getting your steps in is the most important for sleep. Inactivity all day tends to make sleep worse because you are not actually tired. I know I just said no stimulating or intense exercise before bed, but your activity through the remainder of the day makes a difference. Think about how well you sleep after an active day outdoors. The more physical you are, the better you sleep. The second most important exercise besides just walking is squats. Squats are a primal movement that create optimal movement in every joint in your body. Not only that, squats will make you hungrier for the protein you are actually supposed to consume. Many will find that they do not crave or want meat. This is very commonly due to inactivity. If you stress your muscles with exercise, you will want healthier food. You crave it to refuel yourself. I know we always eat more meat on squat days.

Squats

You may be wondering at this point why I talk so much about athletes. That is because HUMANS ARE ATHLETES. All of us. We are meant to move! I do not care if you played sports in high school or not. We are not sedentary beings. We evolved to run and hunt and lift. That is why I try to preach to you to eat like an athlete and to train like one. The first athletic move to master is the Squat.

The squat is the most important movement for life. It is the most dependable indicator for being able to reach old age and still maintain independence and overall health. Think about it. If you lose the ability to get out of a chair without assistance, you quickly gain weight and then have an even harder time moving around and this is a downward spiral toward injury, pain, and misery. That is not to mention that squats protect your joints from injury as well as teach you balance so that you do not experience falls.

Most individuals with ankle, knee, hip or low back pain either cannot perform a squat or they can with extremely improper form. I spoke in earlier chapters about the Paleo chair stretch or yoga squat. This is a great way to start to work on squat mobility. Once you have the mobility, it is time to work on strength and form. Many assume that since they are in pain they need to stop moving. Nothing is farther from the truth. There may be the occasional over-exerciser that needs a rest day or the person recovering from surgery but the vast majority of America does not move enough. The sedentary postures are what causes the pain, the treatment is to move. If squatting causes pain, it is being done incorrectly. A correct squat should not cause pain.

When patients avoid exercise due to pain, they almost always end up worse for the wear. They get weaker and hurt more. Movement inhibits pain. Lack of movement increases it. End of story. I am not saying that you should be able to go straight from couch potato to perfect squat in a week. It takes time. Often, some pain is good when rebuilding. Many people do not know the difference between exercise discomfort and actual pain. This is one circumstance where the "no pain no gain" principle will apply. In order to rebuild a deficiency, some discomfort is needed. That is how we grow. Eventually, this discomfort will decrease overall joint pains and keep you healthier longer.

Learning Progression

If you could read a paragraph to learn squat form this is it. However, I will tell you I am an exercise junkie and I still depend on trainers to make sure I am doing things right. My squat progression starts with squatting to a target. Basically, find a chair and put it a foot or so behind you. Sit down and stand up without using your hands. If this is too hard, find a taller chair. Once you have mastered the chair, do an air squat. This means lean back with your hips, keep your shoulders up and make sure you can see your toes. If your toes disappear, you are too far forward or squatting too deep for your current ability level. Pick a spot on the wall to concentrate on if you are getting wobbly or losing balance. The goal is to get to a point where your hips go just lower than your knee joint. If you have a mirror, be sure your knee stays over the ankle. If they bend in or out too much you can hurt your knees. This extensive description should tell you why you should seek a professional to master the movement. It sounds very complex for something we inherently do correctly at the age of 2.

Of course the squat is not the only magical movement that can improve quality of life, increase bone/muscle mass, and prevent future injuries. Other basic movements to work on are planks, deadlift, pull up, push up, etc. to strengthen the core and back. Usually the ability to perform these movements correctly will eliminate back, hip, knee, ankle, shoulder, and whatever other joint pains.

Weight Bearing

Being able to perform a weighted squat is of utmost importance. This is preferably with a barbell or weighted vest and I will tell you why. It is imperative for overall spinal health to put the spine under load. Applying weight to the shoulders stresses your bones and ligaments in a positive way that causes them to grow. This is called Wolff's Law. It states that a bone will adapt to loads under which it is placed. Muscle growth works the same way. Many of the nutrition protocols discussed in this book will increase bone density. I have seen it in multiple patients whom do not regularly exercise; they start to increase protein and decrease sugars and their bone density tests improve. However, nothing is as effective as putting the spine under load. I highly encourage everyone to join a gym with free weights and hire an instructor to teach you proper mechanics for this movement. You can start with something as simple as your child's book bag to add weight to your squat. Three digit weights are not required to get positive effects.

Assignments:

Get an app or tracker for macros

Create a Bedtime Ritual

Learn to do a barbell squat, hire a coach if needed

The Journey Beyond

I stated at the beginning that the path to wellness is a lifelong journey. Most of us will not reach total health bliss in one year. Life is ever changing. You will always have new stressors and conditions that will affect your body. It is important to consider the lessons learned in this book when new challenges arise. You may need to revisit certain chapters. Different topics will serve you at different points in your life. If you fall off the bandwagon occasionally, try not to let it go to a downward spiral. Instead, revisit a wellness plan that helped you previously and get back into it.

I have fallen off track many, many times. I often need refreshers on these topics I teach so often about. I bounce between protocols based on my life circumstances. There are few occasions where I need help beyond what we have discussed. In these cases, I seek help from other professionals. However, at least 95% of any dysfunction will be remedied by the protocols suggested, the trick is finding the right one at the right time.

For example, I recently got slammed at work. I was working above capacity for a few months straight and eventually paid the price. My adrenals took a dive. I had to go back to that protocol for a month until I felt recovered and confident enough to go back to my high intensity exercise and low carb usual routine. I have done leaky gut protocols more than once. I always watch my sugar. I need reminders to slow life down constantly. Almost every time my health sways from fit and happy to sluggish and low, I revisit the tools here. They bring me back, every time.

Now, what if you did achieve your goals?

When you do reach your initial goals, you must keep moving forward towards new ones. Total fitness is not something you can reach and then quit trying. "Fitness is not owned, it is rented. Rent must be paid daily." Take time to learn something new: try a sport, train for a race, set a body composition goal, etc. Simply ask yourself, "What is my best life? What does it look like?" If there is something missing, set action steps to get it. Taking time to meditate on what your happiest you looks like will also bring about change via the Law of Attraction.

Law of Attraction

"Be the energy you want to attract in the world!"

I know for some this seems like a bunch of hum bug but it is a long time proven principle of the universe. Whether you call it prayer, affirmations, energy, intention, or whatever, it does have some merit. The law of attraction is the principle that if you can truly believe something will happen and want it bad enough, it will happen. It shows that negative thoughts lead to negative outcomes and positive ones lead to positive outcomes. Obviously there are limitations to this as we cannot perform miracles or control the lives of others. However, we can control our own destiny and outcomes.

I will tell you that I found my husband as a direct result of the law of attraction. I always wanted to marry this magical version of a man. He would be a fit country boy, intelligent, kind mannered, motivated, like horses and camping and mountaineering, snowboard, and on top of all that he would respect that I am a driven career women. Can you believe I found all of these attributes? I did not have to compromise a single one. When I first met Travis I assumed he was from Alabama or something with his gentlemanly presentation, good manner and slight accent. He was actually from Ohio, but a country boy nonetheless. Now here is where the law of attraction gets tricky. It is not magic; you cannot just sit around waiting for things. You must take action to get what you want. So how did I find what I wanted? I put myself in an environment with likeminded people and above all I worked on myself. Prior to meeting Travis, I had started Crossfit. I got super healthy and fit (not skinny mind you, just fit) and mostly just hung out with my gym peeps. I had sworn to be single for a year to work on myself. That is when he walked into my gym before starting his first semester at Chiropractic School.

So let's recap the things I did to work on myself that brought him to me. I went to college, got into graduate school, joined clubs at school that introduced me to Crossfit, I got really serious about lifting, did some competitions, stuck with my resolutions for almost a year, and then met him. No, the law of attraction is not magic. It just shows that working towards something relentlessly will eventually manifest what you want most. I became the example of the life I wanted to achieve and the man I wanted to meet. By working towards something, I opened up opportunities to find a better life. Another way to be the example and attract better things is to teach it. Travis and I were both Crossfit coaches.

Teaching is the best way to become a master and stay accountable.

The best way to maintain your health and reach your goals is to teach others. Have you ever heard of the principle that states: if you can teach others, you learn the material better yourself? It is so true. I encourage you to find a way to spread your newfound wellness knowledge. Now this doesn't mean you have to go get a Master's or a Doctorate. Find something you love. Learn to teach yoga or spinning. Coach a team. Start teaching workshops. Become a health coach.

We all love to hate on the pyramid scheme type supplements and workout companies. However, if you do have a company that resonates with you, it can be very helpful for staying healthy. I was a Beach body coach while in school. I learned a great deal about motivation and accountability while doing this job. My friends still involved in this company are fitter than they ever were in our younger years. It keeps them going because they have some skin in the game. They have to stay fit to keep their business going. They coach others to become and stay fit as well and that helps their ongoing motivation.

If you make health your career in some way shape or form you will have the accountability to stick with your journey. Most class instructors stay fit. If you think of your generic gym; there are a multitude of workout classes taught by the average Joe. You can earn a weekend certificate in things like spinning and barbell blast. I earned my Crossfit Level 1 over a weekend and was able to coach Crossfit to pay off my membership when I first started my Chiropractic practice. It was a great way to make exercise affordable. I also became better at my sport because I was teaching it. I now coach high school tennis. It forces me to stay on top of my game. It also brings me great joy to teach the game to the students. Find something in your life that helps you teach while staying accountable.

Final Thoughts

Teaching you all via this book has definitely brought more accountability to my life. I appreciate the opportunity to help you, which in turn has helped me greatly as well. I thank you all for your time and effort. I honor your decision to create a better you, or simply recreate a past you that was vibrant and healthy. Knowing how health is a constant struggle to maintain, I applaud you for making it this far without giving up! It is a true attestation to your strength and vitality. May you continue through your journey towards an optimal existence. May you find all the happiness you deserve. May help always arise when you most need it. Namaste.

Appendix

Gluten Ingredients 229

High Likelihood Gluten Contamination 230

Gluten Cross Reactors 231

Caster Oil Packs 232

Coffee Enemas 233

SIBO Food Protocol 237

Moderate Fasting Protocol 238

Adrenal Fatigue Protocol 240

Detox Protocol 243

Leaky Gut Protocol 244

Macro Lists 246

Paleo Shopping List 249

Keto Shopping List 250

Inflammation Factors 251

Glycemic Index 252

Gluten Ingredients

Here is a list of where gluten may be hidden:Barley (flakes, flour, pearl)

Breading, bread stuffing

Brewer's yeast

Bulgur

Durum (type of wheat)

Farro/faro (also known as spelt or dinkel)

Graham flour

Hydrolyzed wheat protein

Kamut (type of wheat)

Malt, malt extract, malt syrup, malt flavoring

Malt vinegar

Malted milk

Matzo, matzo meal

Modified wheat starch

Oatmeal, oat bran, oat flour, whole oats (unless they are from pure, uncontaminated oats)

Rye bread and flour

Seitan (a meat-like food derived from wheat gluten used in many vegetarian dishes)

Semolina

Spelt (type of wheat also known as farro, faro, or dinkel)

Triticale

Wheat bran

Wheat flour

Wheat germ

Wheat starch

Atta (chapati flour)

Einkorn (type of wheat)

Emmer (type of wheat)

High Likelihood of Gluten Contamination:

Beer, ale, lager

Breads

Broth, soup, soup bases

Cereals

Cookies and crackers

Some chocolates, some chocolate bars, licorice

Flavored coffees and teas

Imitation bacon bits, imitation seafood

Medications (check with your pharmacist)

Gluten Cross Reactors

Processed foods

Salad dressings

Sausages, hot dogs, deli meats

Sauces, marinades, gravies

Seasonings

Soy sauce

Shampoo, conditioners, lotions, make-up

Amaranth

Barley

Buckwheat

Chocolate

Coffee

Corn

Dairy, i.e. milk and cheese (alpha-casein, beta-casein, casomorphin, butyrophilin, whey protein)

Egg

Hemp

Millet

Oats

Polish wheat

Potato

Rye

Rice

Sesame

Spelt

Sorghum

Soy

Tapioca

Teff

Yeast

These lists are very overwhelming. I suggest getting a phone app that you can use to scan grocery items such as InRFood, Food Intolerances, or find me gluten free. That or simply avoid all grains and processed food.

Castor oil pack instructions

Need: Cotton Wool, Hot pack/pad, Plastic Barrier, Caster Oil

1. Make a pack approximately the size of your hand. (Cut a piece of cotton wool and soak it with 2 tbsp. of castor oil or until saturated.

2. Position pack over liver (under right breast tissue). Packs may be used on other body areas for detox as well if you have a part of interest. Put plastic over the pack to protect oil from ruining your hot pack. Beware oil will stain. May be helpful to wear old clothes or towels.

3. Place hot pack on top of plastic. Be careful not to burn yourself! Do not fall asleep with pack on.

4. Allow pack to remain for 15 min at first. Some people can handle more time than others but it's advisable to gradually increase time with each application. You may go up to 1 hour. Too much time on first application may leave you feeling pretty beat.

5. You may use pack daily for 2-3 weeks although this length is not required for results. Many will notice detox in the form of altered bowel motility or grogginess followed by clarity. Many other results are possible.

6. Cleaning may require baking soda if excess is still on skin or appliances.

COFFEE ENEMA INSTRUCTION

What many envision when I say coffee enema is something similar to a colonoscopy. That is NOT the case. Coffee enemas are minimally invasive and require little money. They can be done on your own in the privacy of your own bathroom. Many shutter at the idea of starting this practice. However, I encourage you to give it a try. It is not as uncomfortable as most imagine and can offer amazing results with just one application. This therapy has implications in cancer therapy, detox, gut disorders such as SIBO, as well as simply clearing the gut of unwanted material. Coffee enema benefits include hydrating the colon, cleansing the colon, stimulating bile flow, and enhanced detox to the liver. It is well known in the Gerson Therapy for cancer and that is the protocol followed here.

I recommend the Pure Life Coffee Enema kit, however, materials may be found at your local pharmacy usually. It provides all needed materials (besides a coffee maker).

Materials

Organic Coffee, Enema Bucket or bag (2 qtr.), long plastic tube with applicator, water, lemon

How Often

Coffee Enemas can be done as many times as 6 per day or as little as once a year. They are a good practice to add for your health either way. Your doctor may give you a better indication of how often you may benefit from this procedure.

Best Time

The best time is after a normal bowel movement, at home, and in a relaxed environment. It may be wise to not perform them in the evening due to a slight caffeine rush.

Preparation

It is helpful, especially if you have not had a movement or are constipated, to do a lemon water cleanse first. This is simply done by squeezing a lemon into 2 cups of water. Do not use cold water. Room temp up to body temp are good temperatures. Apply this liquid through the apparatus first to cleanse colon and hopefully induce a movement. This should make holding the coffee easier. The lemon water will likely not be held long, if you last 5 minutes that is plenty and you can use the toilet. After this you may move onto the coffee portion.

- BOILING METHOD - Place 2 to 3 cups of **purified water** and **two to three tablespoons of coffee** in a saucepan and bring to a boil (or use a coffee maker). Let it boil 5 minutes, then turn off the heat and allow it to cool. One or two ice cubes may be added to speed the cooling process. You may make a larger quantity and use it for several enemas. Wait until the water is **comfortable to the touch.** If the water is too hot or too cold, retaining the enema will be more difficult. Strain the liquid through a fine strainer or coffee filter paper into a clean enema bag. Screw on the top of the enema bag. The enema is now ready.

- PREPARE CONTAINER HOSES - Be sure the plastic hose is pushed or fastened well onto the enema bag and the thin enema tip is attached to the other end

-REMOVE AIR - Remove any air from the enema tube the following way. Grasp but do not close the clamp on the hose. Place the tip in the sink. Hold up the enema bag above the tip until the water begins to flow out. Then close the clamp. This expels any air in the tube.

-LUBRICATE - Lubricate the enema tip with a small amount of soap or oil. We like to use coconut oil. (Too much lubrication will cause the tip to fall out of the rectum, creating a mess!).

TAKING THE ENEMA

- POSITION - The position preferred by most people is lying on one's back on a towel, on the bathroom floor or in the bathtub. An alternative is sitting on the toilet, which does not give as much gravity feed. This also makes it more difficult to hold. It is best to start on left side lying, then go to back, then to the right side in order to spread coffee through colon.

- PLACE CONTAINER ABOVE - With the clamp closed, hang the bag about one foot above your abdomen.

- INSERT - Insert the tip gently and slowly. Move it around until it goes all the way in.

- OPENFLOW - Open the clamp and hold the enema bag about one foot above the abdomen. The water may take a few seconds to begin flowing. If the water does not flow, you may gently squeeze the bag. If you develop a cramp, close the hose clamp, turn from side to side and take a few deep breaths. The cramp will usually pass quickly.

- WHEN FULL -When all the liquid is inside, the bag will become flat or the container will be empty. Close the clamp. You can leave the tube inserted, or remove it slowly. It is beneficial to massage liquid through (up left abdomen, across upper, and down right). Keeping firm pressure on tender points for a few seconds may help cramps.

- RETAIN THE ENEMA FOR up to 15 MINUTES – Two 7 min sessions can be effective if your bowel does not allow full enema yet. A coffee Enema is an exercise for your gut musculature, it may require some conditioning before you are good at it. You may remain lying on the floor. Use the time to read a book, meditate, etc. Some people are able to get up and go lie on a towel in bed, instead of on the floor. Walking around the house with the coffee inside is not recommended.

FINISHING UP

After 15 minutes or so, go to the toilet and empty out the water. It is okay if some water remains inside. If water remains inside often, you are dehydrated.

- WASH EQUIPMENT - Wash the enema bag or container and tube thoroughly.

Coffee Enema Protocol From:

The Little Enema Book from purelifeenema.com and the Gerson Therapy

SIBO Food Protocol

Foods to eat

Protein-chicken, fish, eggs

Nuts-all nuts accept pistachios

Low fructose fruit- apricots, avocado, cantaloupe, grapefruit, honeydew melon, nectarine, orange, peach, pineapple, raspberries, strawberries, tomato

Low fructan (fructose polymer) vegetables-bamboo shoot, bell pepper, bok choy, broccoli, carrots, celery, chard, chilies, chives, choy sum, courgettes, cucumbers, endive, fennel, ginger, kale, olives, parsnips, parsley, pumpkins, radishes, rutabaga, spinach, squash, turnips, zucchini

Fats-animal fats, oils

Foods to avoid

Protein: Beef, lamb, pork

Sugar: natural and artificial sweeteners (honey, agave, stevia, sorbitol, mannitol, xylitol, etc.), anything made with corn syrup

Grain: all wheat products, all gluten free grains (amaranth, quinoa, millet, buckwheat, tapioca, etc.), all corn products (cornstarch, corn flour, cornmeal etc.), rice

Legumes/galactans: beans, chickpeas, lentils, peas, soybeans

Dairy Products (lactose and Casein): all milk and whey sources

High Fructan (fructose polymers) Vegetables: artichokes, asparagus, beets, brussel sprouts, cabbage, cauliflower, green peppers, lettuce, mushrooms, okra, onion, peas, shallots

High-Starch vegetables- plantains, potatoes, sweet potatoes, yucca

High Fructose Fruit- apples, bananas, blueberries, cherries, grapes, kiwi, mango, watermelon

Moderate Fasting Instruction

(Insulin Resistance Protocol)

Ingredients

Lemon/lime Juice Fresh Squeezed

Organic Maple Syrup (grade b preferred)

Bone Broth

Spring Water

Green tea optional

Please be aware that if you have hypoglycemic tendencies, this may not be the right approach for you. To monitor yourself, you may buy a blood glucose monitor from any pharmacy. Try to be sure that your glucose stays under 100 and above 80.

Phase 1

Fill one gallon of water with 2 tsp maple syrup and juice of 1 lemon (fresh brewed green tea optional.) Drink this throughout the day (ratio of ingredients may be altered). It should be sipped on every ten to fifteen minutes to keep blood sugar stable. Drinking a lot at a time or going long periods between drinks will not reach the desired effect. Meals may be replaced with any bone broth or collagen. This "diet" should be continued for at least three days, up to 20 depending on your resolve. I will also note that it is most beneficial to do a water only fast but I know this is not possible for certain hypoglycemic individuals.

Phase 2

After the juice phase, choose 1 vegetable, one fat, and one meat to consume for the next few days. Each subsequent day 1 food may be added. The slower/longer the process, the better. Eating strict for at least three weeks is optimal.

For optimal digestive health it is necessary to have fruit, vegetables, meat, sweet potato, and coconut as your primary foods. Other foods may affect you negatively to varying degrees. Be careful how quickly you re-introduce certain foods as they may cause digestive irritation after your stomach accommodating to very little food.

Phase 3

Gradually add in more foods. Be mindful of what you can tolerate. Carbohydrates should not make you sleepy, if they do you ate too many and spiked your insulin too much. Anything that causes gas/bloating is to be eliminated.

Phase 4

Entire system may be repeated after 1 month.

Adrenal Fatigue Protocol

This is for those looking to stabilize blood sugar that struggle with hypoglycemia or adrenal burn out. There are 10 steps to implement.

1-Avoid the middle isles

Middle isle food (anything boxed, canned, bagged or frozen is likely loaded with dangerous additives. The most common additive is high fructose corn syrup. Fructose is responsible for a high blood sugar spikes and subsequent insulin response. This sugar creates a lot of blood sugar instability.

2- Eat every 2-3 hours.

This means breakfast and second breakfast and even bedtime snacks! Eating within an hour of waking is a way to tell your body that it is not in starvation mode it was the past 12 hours you were fasting/sleeping. Eating a hearty breakfast is a great way to jumpstart your metabolism and give you something to burn off through the day. Food is fuel! YOU cannot expect your body to perform with no logs on the fire. The 200 calorie smoothie for breakfast burns off very quickly. I suggest eating at minimum 600 calories between first and second breakfast. If you are prevented from eating in the morning due to no hunger or nausea, you may need to start slowly in order to reset your biological clock or see a physician that can help you with digestion. Note: The more you eat earlier in the day, the less you will feel like binging on sugar at dinner time.

3-Eat more fat

Your metabolism is like a fire. Without any logs on the fire you will not keep a stable blood sugar throughout the day. Fats have been the root of all criticism the past few decades. However, your body was not made with spare parts. You have lipase to break it down in the digestive tract for a reason. Don't get me wrong, there are poor sources of fat. Trans fats in fried foods and potato chips causes and immense amount of inflammation in the body. However, MUFA's, mono-unsaturated fats, are great for just the opposite. These are found in foods like avocado, olive oil, and olives. These are fabulous for stabilizing blood sugar by including them with each meal. Fats hardly have a glycemic index (aka insulin response) like carbohydrates. Fat also induces the fullness response to the brain after eating. Sugar inhibits this response and causes you to eat more and more. Omega-3's in flaxseed and fish help decrease inflammation as well as stabilize sugars. Omega-3s can actually reduce pain through similar pathways as ibuprofen.

4-Get your inflammation level down

You like sugar, so does cancer, diabetes, insomnia, yeast. Arthritis, and inflammation. Besides balancing blood sugar, inflammation is decreased by eating a high veggie Paleolithic diet, adding omega-3, taking turmeric, and reducing stress.

5-Avoid Stimulants

Stimulants inhibit your appetite by mobilizing glucose into the bloodstream. When they wear off, you want to binge out on sugary foods to bring your blood glucose back up. Stimulants do this by stimulating your adrenal glands (the ones that help you deal with stress) to secrete cortisol and catecholamines. With chronic use of stimulants, the adrenals get tired of always trying to secrete these substances so they stop or slow down. This leads to further blood sugar dysregulation because cortisol is needed to get glucose into the bloodstream when you have not eaten.

6- Moderate exercise

Vigorous exercise can be detrimental to an already fatigued adrenal gland. The best exercise is long mild cardio (such as walking or biking), to a point that you can still speak or sing while doing it. Depending on the level of adrenal burn out, it may be best to avoid all exercise besides yoga. A good way to determine if you exercise too vigorous is how you feel after. If exercise causes a need for a nap or coffee, it is too hard.

7-Reduce stress

Meditation and yoga are the obvious suggestions for reducing stress. See later chapters for more info on these. A less obvious suggestion would be to eliminate stress from your life. This could be radical, such as quitting a job or ending a relationship. The important thing is that quitting a bad relationship or job may prolong your life. So as radical as it may seem, drastic action may be necessary.

8-Avoid food allergies

Allergies are a form of stimulant on the body. All stimulants must be avoided to heal the adrenals.

9-Sleep often and enough

Getting 6-8 hours of sleep is for good health. However, when recovering the adrenals much more than this may be necessary, even taking naps!

10-Find joy every day!

Detox Program Food (21 days recommended)

Foods to avoid:

•Any food that you are allergic to it. •Dairy (milk, cheese, yogurt, butter), eggs, margarine, and shortening •Foods prepared with Gluten containing cereals like wheat, oats, rye, barley, normally found in breads, pasta, etc. •Tomatoes and tomato sauces, corn, peanuts •Alcohol, Caffeine (coffee, black tea, sodas) •Soy or products made from soy, such soy milk or tofu •Peanuts or peanut butter• Beef, pork, cold cuts, bacon, hotdogs, canned meat, sausage, shellfish, meat analogues made from soy

Foods to eat:

•Drink plenty of water (8-10 glasses), herbal teas, green tea, fruit juices (no sugar added), vegetable juices •Consume grain foods made from rice, millet, quinoa, buckwheat or tapioca. •Fresh fruits, vegetables, beans (navy, white, red kidney, etc., peas (fresh, split, snap) •Consume mainly fish (not shellfish), and moderate amounts of chicken, turkey, and lamb •Use mainly olive oil, canola and flax seed oil in moderation

Leaky Gut Food Protocol

Food to eat:

Most organic Vegetables: Anise, artichokes, asparagus, beets, bok choy, broccoli, cabbage, carrots, cauliflower, celery, chives, cucumbers, garlic, kale, kohlrabi, leeks, lettuce, mustard greens, onions, parsley, radish, rhubarb, shallots, spinach, squash, sweet potato, water chestnuts, watercress, yams, zucchini.

Low glycemic Fruit: apples, apricots, avocados, berries, cherries, grapefruit, grape, lemon, orange, peach, pear, plum

Meat: beef, chicken, wild caught fish, lamb, turkey. Select hormone free, grass fed, and antibiotic free.

Fermented food: kimchi, kombucha, pickled ginger, sauerkraut, unsweet coconut yogurt.

Coconut: coconut butter, coconut oil, coconut milk, coconut cream, unsweet coconut flakes.

Noodles: brown shirataki yam noodles

Herbs and spices: basil, cilantro, coriander, cumin, curry, garlic, ginger, lemongrass, mint, oregano, parsley, rosemary, sage, sea salt, thyme.

Other: apple cider vinegar, herbal tea, olive oil, olives.

Food to moderate or avoid:

Sugars: agave, candy, chocolate, corn syrup, fructose, high fructose corn syrup and artificial sweeteners, honey, maple syrup, molasses, sucrose.

High glycemic fruits: bananas, canned fruits, dried fruit, mango, pineapple, raisins, watermelon.

Grains: amaranth, barley, buckwheat, bulgur wheat, corn, couscous, kamut, millet, oats, quinoa, rice, rye, spelt, wheat, wheat germ.

Gluten containing food: BBQ sauce, binders, bouillon, brewer's yeast, cold cuts, condiments, emulsifiers, fillers, chewing gum, hot dogs, hydrolyzed plant or vegetable protein, ketchup, soy sauce, lunch meats, malt, matzo, modified food starch, monosodium glutamate, non dairy creamer (I am not talking about almond/coconut milk), processed salad dressings, seitan, some spice mixes, teriyaki sauce, textured vegetable protein.

Dairy products and eggs: butter, cheese, cow's milk, cream, frozen desserts, goats milk, margarine, sheep's milk, mayonnaise, whey, and yogurt.

Soy: edamame, miso, soy milk, soy protein, soy sauce, tempeh, tofu.

Alcohol: all alcohol.

Beans and legumes: black beans, lentils, peanuts, pinto beans, soybeans.

Nuts and seeds: almonds, peanuts, sunflower seeds, sesame seeds.

Nightshade foods: eggplant, paprika, peppers, potatoes, hot sauce, tomatillos, tomatoes.

Fungi: edible fungi and mushrooms.

Macro List

Chart of Favorable Macros (80%)

Protein (cooked)	Favorable Carb (cooked)	Favorable Carb (raw)	Fats (for 1.5g)	Fruits (favorable carbs)
Beef	Artichoke	Broccoli	Almonds	Apple
Calamari	Asparagus	Cabbage	Avocado	Applesauce
Ham/ Bacon	Black Beans	Carrot	Bacon Bits	Apricots
Canned Tuna	Broccoli	Cauliflower	Butter	Blackberries
Catfish	Brussels Sprouts	Celery	Cashews	Blueberries
Cheese	Cabbage	Cucumber	Coconut Oil	Cantaloupe
Chicken Breast	Cauliflower	Lettuce	Cream Cheese	Cherries
Clams	ChickPeas	Mushrooms	Guacamole	Grapefruit
Corned Beef	Dill Pickles	Onion	Half and Half	Grapes
Cottage Cheese	Eggplant	Peppers	Lard	Honeydew
Crabmeat	Green Beans	Radishes	Macadamia Nuts	Kiwi
Deli-meat	Kale	Salsa	Mayonnaise	Lemon
Duck	Kidney Beans	Spinach	Olive Oil	Lime
Ground Beef	Leeks	Tomato	Olives	Nectarine
Ground Lamb	Lentils	Zucchini	Peanut Butter	Orange
Ground Pork	Oatmeal	Sprouts	Peanuts	Peach
Ground Turkey	Okra	Peas	Salad Dressing	Pear
Lamb	Onion		Sesame Oil	Pineapple

Lobster	Sauerkraut		Sour Cream	Plum
Pork	Spaghetti Squash		Sunflower Seeds	Raspberries
Protein Powder	Spinach		Tahini	Strawberries
Salmon	Tomato Sauce		Tartar Sauce	Tangerine
Sardines	Tomatoes		Walnuts	Watermelon
Scallops	Yellow Squash		Coconut Milk	
Seitan	Zucchini		Coconut Flakes	
Shrimp	Greens			
swordfish	Sweet potato			
Tuna Steak	Turnips			
Turkey Breast	Parsnips			
Veal	Squash			
Egg	Carrots			
	Beets			

Chart of Less Favorable Carbohydrates (20%)

Vegetables	Fruit	Grains and Bread	Condiments	Alcohol	Snacks
Baked Beans	Banana	Bagel	BBQ Sauce	Beer	Chocolate Bar
Black Eyed Peas	Cranberries	Biscuit	Brown Sugar	Liquor	Corn Chips
Corn	Cranberry Sauce	Bread	Ketchup	Wine	Graham Crackers
French Fries	Dates	Bread Crumbs	Cocktail Sauce		Ice Cream
Lima Beans	Figs	Bread Sticks	Confectioners' Sugar		Potato Chips
Peas	Guava	Cereal	Granulated Sugar		Pretzels
Pinto Beans	Kumquat	Corn Bread	Honey		Saltine Crackers
White Potatoes	Mango	Croissant	Jelly/Jam		Tortilla Chips
Potatoes	Papaya	Crouton	Maple Syrup		
Refried Beans	Prunes	Doughnut	Molasses		
	Raisins	English Muffin	Pickle (bread & butter)		
		Flour	Plum Sauce		
		Granola	Relish		
		Grits	Steak Sauce		
		Instant Oatmeal	Teriyaki Sauce		
		Muffins			
		Noodles			
		Pancake			
		Pasta			

Dr. Rachel Brooks

Paleo Shopping List

Proteins:
Beef
Fish
Chicken
Eggs
Duck
Venison
Elk
Bison
Seafood
Turkey
Pork

Fats:
Coconut oil
Olive Oil
Nut Oils
Animal Fats
Butter

Fruit:
Berries
Green Apples
Olives
Avocado
Melon
Tomatoes
Coconut
Lemon/Lime

Starch:
Sweet Potato
Parsnips

Radish
Beets
Rutabaga
Turnips
Carrots
Squash

Vegetables:
Green Leafy
Broccoli
Cauliflower
Asparagus
Onions
Brussels sprouts
Artichoke
Cucumber
Spaghetti Squash
Zucchini

Baking:
Almond Flour
Cassava Flour
Baking
(Soda/Powder)
Dark   Chocolate
(80% or more)
Maple Syrup
Honey

*Miscellaneous:
Mushrooms
Condiments
Vinegars

Spices
Coconut Aminos
Almond Milk
Coconut
Milk/Cream
Teas
Coffee
Club Soda
*All items must be
sugar freeLard
Avocado Oil
Grapeseed
Ghee
Tapioca Flour
Coconut Flour

Keto Shopping List

Proteins:

Beef

Fish

Chicken

Eggs

Duck

Venison

Elk

Bison

Seafood

Turkey

Pork

Cheese

Fats:

Coconut oil

Olive Oil

Nut Oils

Animal Fats

Butter

Lard

Avocado Oil

Grapeseed

Ghee

Heavy Cream

Sugar Free Dairy

Fruit:

Olives

Avocado

Tomatoes

Coconut

Lemon/Lime

Vegetables:

Green Leafy

Broccoli

Cauliflower

Asparagus

Onions

Brussels sprouts

Cucumber

Spaghetti Squash

Zucchini

Baking:

Almond Flour

Coconut Flour

Baking

(Soda/Powder)

Dark   Chocolate

(80% or more)

*Miscellaneous:

Mushrooms

Condiments

Vinegars

Spices

Coconut Aminos

Almond Milk

Coconut

Milk/Cream

Teas

Coffee

Club Soda

*All items must be

sugar free

FACTORS THAT AFFECT INFLAMMATION

Increase Pain

Decrease Pain

Diet

Increase Pain
- Excess sugar + carbohydrates
- Soda
- Drugs/Smoking/Alcohol
- Too much **BAD FATS**
- Crash Diets/ Severely low-fat diets
- Dehydration

Decrease Pain
- Omega 3 Foods
- Protein rich diet (30% Daily Intake)
- Balance Macros (40, 30, 30)
- Eating appropriate calories (not under or over) Lots of dark colored fruits/vegetables high

Lifestyle

Increase Pain
- Lack of exercise
- Lack of mobility
- Lack of human interaction
- Over-exercise
- Toxic work environment (emotional or chemical)

Decrease Pain
- Exercise
- Play
- Good sleep
- Good hygiene

Emotional

Increase Pain
- Loss of support systems
- Not feeling appreciated
- Depression
- Excessive stress

Decrease Pain
- Joining community groups
- Connect w/ Family/friends
- Choose to forget bad relationships
- Find a job/hobby that creates fulfillment

Structural

Increase Pain
- Lack of spinal movement
- Uneven muscle contracture
- Injury
- Illness

Decrease Pain
- Yoga
- Massage
- Chiropractic
- Laser Therapy
- Acupuncture

Other

Increase Pain
- Eating too fast
- Infection
- Allergies
- Indigestion
- Underlying disease

Decrease Pain
- Slow down diet
- Enzymes

Glycemic Index

High

Cereal	Dark Rice
White breads	Ice Cream
White Flours	Pineapple
Cereal	Cantaloupe
Juice	**Low**
Sport Drinks	Other fruit
Soda	Vegetables
White Potato	Dairy
White Rice	Agave
Snack Foods	Maple
Splenda	Coconut
Moderate	Nuts
Popcorn	Corn
Dried Fruit	Alcohol
Honey	Oats
Table Sugar	Sweet Potato
Whole Grains	

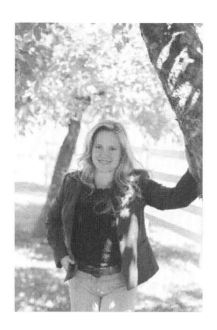

About The Author

Dr. Rachel Brooks is a Chiropractor in Fort Gratiot, MI. She graduated from Logan University with her Doctorate in Chiropractic and Master's in Nutrition after earning her Bachelor's in Microbiology from the University of Michigan. She owns a practice with her husband, Dr. Travis Tourjee and also works with her sisters that specialize in massage and nutrition as well. Dr. Rachel enjoys walks/hikes with her dog Stella, Crossfit with her hubby, coffee dates with family, traveling, and days at the lake in Michigan.

Made in the USA
Lexington, KY
05 August 2019